IMPROVE YOUR MOOD WITH FOOD

FOODS THAT FIGHT DEPRESSION

Alexandra Massey

with Anita Bean

Publisher's warning: if you are currently undergoing a course
of prescribed medication for depression, we strongly advise that
you do not stop taking it without first consulting your GP.

First published in The United States in 2006 by
Virgin Books Ltd
Thames Wharf Studios
Rainville Road
London
W6 9HA

First Published in Great Britain in 2006 by Virgin Books Ltd

A catalogue record for this book is available from the British Library.

ISBN 0 7535 1192 4
9 7807535 1192 3

Designed by seagulls

Printed in Peru

Contents

Introduction

I have always had a difficult relationship with food. As far back as I can remember I have eaten food based on how I'm feeling. From the age of five or six I used to sneak into the cupboard and pinch some of my dad's chocolate cookies if I felt bad. From the age of nine onward I must have been aware of how body shape mattered because I would put myself on a diet and tell everyone about it; maybe I wanted to be like an adult or perhaps I needed some attention. Whatever the case, I had a push-pull affiliation with food that became more intense the older I got. It was only when I took stock of what was happening to me and began to recognize the improvements that could be made to my sense of wellbeing from eating more healthily that I could change my habits. I began to notice that a day of healthy eating would mean I had much more energy, uplifting my overall outlook; conversely, a day of junk food with sugary snacks and high-fat meals meant I was more likely to wake up the next day feeling tired, depressed and fed up.

We all use food and drink as a way of changing our mood. Look at the way we use coffee to get us going in the morning, a bar of chocolate as a treat, or a glass of champagne to help us celebrate. Using food to change the way we feel is embedded in our eating culture. *Top Santé* magazine found that 61 percent of us would rather have a good meal than a night of passion. Food is the way we can comfort ourselves, offer ourselves an indulgence, or pamper someone with a sumptuous feast.

However, the foods we eat to cheer ourselves up are often "quick fixes" that come with a downside. Foods such as cakes and cookies deposit large amounts of sugar into the bloodstream. This provides a quick energy boost but then the fall in blood sugar sometime afterwards can be accompanied by tiredness, a low mood and even dizziness and shaking. Although our bodies make us aware of such symptoms, we rarely associate them with low blood-sugar levels or with what we ate earlier. We tend instead to put these feelings down to "fatigue" or "stress."

Nevertheless, there is an increasing amount of research pointing toward food as having a powerful effect on the way we feel, both physically and emotionally. As this is a relatively new field, there aren't a lot of definites, but there is a certainty that if you eat the right food at the right time your chemistry will be balanced, which will make you feel great; eat the wrong food at the wrong time and this may cause insomnia, stress, exacerbated PMT and general fatigue, and leave your immune system vulnerable to attack from cold and flu viruses. In a recent survey of 200 people carried out by the "Food & Mood Project," run by MIND, 88 percent said that changing their diet for the better significantly improved their mood.

Of course there are many other factors that can affect our disposition, such as our financial security, home life or relationships at work, but the exciting thing about the food/mood link is that it opens up a whole new world of knowledge at our fingertips. Rather than wondering why we feel so tired, considering a visit to the doctor or berating ourselves for not feeling better, we actually have some of the answers in our own kitchen. The fact that we can plan our meals in accordance with the way we would like to feel is liberating. Not only that, but the time needed to feel the difference in our physical and emotional wellbeing can be as little as a matter of hours.

This book will look at ways of eating that can dramatically enhance our emotional wellbeing together with two straightforward concepts to streamline good eating habits: the "Five-a-Day" rule and "Three Meals a Day." It also offers food for thought by looking at ten areas of modern behavior around eating and offers top tips that can be easily assimilated into a busy life.

We also take a look at "Emotional Eating," of which there has been a huge increase in recent years. Emotional Eating is the practice of stifling negative feelings through eating comforting food. According to new research, a quarter of us eat when we are stressed and at least 40 percent of us eat when we are bored. This can set up a vicious circle. For example, if we want to ignore an emotion that is nagging at us, and we comfort ourselves by eating sugary or fatty foods, we can end up feeling physically and emotionally worse than we did originally. The good news is that "emotional eaters" do not actually consume more than non-emotional eaters when in stressful situations; it's just that they generally indulge in foods that are higher in fat and calories. In this book, we look at the key to re-educating our taste buds, learning to equate emotional wellbeing with new tastes and flavors. This is not as difficult as it may sound. Contrary to popular belief, foods that produce good moods can also be delicious.

We don't have to eat foods we don't enjoy in order to feel better. A steady introduction of good-mood foods into the kitchen can change our bodies' cravings quite quickly—even to the point where we will begin to hanker after the stuff that will make us feel better. We will begin to feel less enamored by the sugary, salty and high-fat foods. When introduced to delicious good-mood foods that are effortless to prepare, you might wonder why you haven't tried them before. Sometimes it's as simple as trying one new recipe to set you off onto a new course of action. The recipes in this book present a range of foods and flavors to tantalize the palate, while at the same time offering a nutritional base for feeling great.

We will look at the top five areas of the modern diet to which the experts draw our attention because they have the most powerfully negative influence on the way we look and feel. It is often perplexing trying to find the right solution to changing our eating habits due to information overload about what we should and shouldn't be eating. *Improve Your Mood*

With Food will also explain the top ten bad-food fallouts by giving some straightforward facts and incorporating simple recommendations for improvements that will begin to take effect almost immediately.

This said, a little of what we fancy can do us the power of good. We can't underestimate the enjoyment of the occasional extravagance. A little luxury can bring an enormous sense of pleasure, but our indulgences need not be unhealthy: a spoon of honey onto nutty-tasting wholemeal bread, some roasted almonds and sunflower seeds or a deliciously creamy houmous that children will dip into with chopped vegetables are just some of the recipes included in the book.

I have got together with award-winning nutritionist Anita Bean to get the best possible recipes with the best mood-food results. This is a resource for anyone who wants recipes and ideas for great-tasting, mood-lifting meals. You can use the book to help plan your diet according to how you want to feel. It is a guide for people who want to feel better through what they eat. It is also designed to clarify some of the negative facts and figures that we read about the food you eat and to offer alternative strategies to help you to look and feel better. You will be surprised and delighted at the variety of foods that can be uplifting and energizing.

Read, eat and enjoy!

1
HOW DO
YOU FEEL?

If you were to just stop for a moment to evaluate exactly how you feel, would your response include any of these?

Full of the joys of spring
Vibrant
Full of enthusiasm
Brimming with energy
Happy to be alive
Enjoying the moment
Loving the people around me
Relaxed and happy

Or would your response include one of these descriptions?

Depressed and grumpy
Stressed out
Anxious and overloaded
Angry and fed up
Feel like crying
Always tired . . .
. . . But can't sleep well
Can't be bothered
Don't know what's wrong with me

There is a powerful link between what we eat and the way we feel. The type of food we eat can have an influential effect on our emotions. We have a firm grasp on "we are what we eat" but science is only just turning its head toward understanding that our food can affect our mood.

Whilst researching for this book I spoke to many people, friends, colleagues, family, etc., of whom at least 70 percent said, "Do you really think that the two are linked?" or "Surely food can't make you feel depressed—surely not?" The idea that food and mood, but particularly depression, are linked is met with reticence and disbelief, but the figures that are coming out prove otherwise.

From my own personal experience, I know that when I have a day of bad-mood food: a picnic (which may include chips and other salty foods, barbecues and white bread with not much fiber and lots of sugary snacks), or food "on the run" (sandwich and a coffee), or by grabbing a processed meal and throwing it in the oven, I can feel depressed, down and miserable the following day. Conversely, when I have a day of balanced meals, wholesome, loving foods and little or no sugar, I will feel great the following day—fully alive, buoyant and with a spring in my step.

For decades so much advice from the experts has covered eating healthily for general good health, especially for the heart and obesity, but there is little informed data pointing toward a diet to make you feel happy. Yet the World Health Organization states that by 2020, on current trends, depression will become the number one health problem, overtaking heart disease and obesity. The American Psychiatric Association reports that 10 percent of the population in the US are depressed at any one time and that's just according to the numbers of people who register with doctors for antidepressants. There has been a 253 percent rise in antidepressant-prescribing in the last ten years, yet, according to a paper published in the *American Journal of Psychiatry* in November 2004, placebos can be as effective as antidepressants in some cases. The question is: where else can we look to find a way to beat depression?

THE HAPPINESS/ FOOD CONNECTION

Food, like a lover's touch, can comfort and seduce us. Paradise is a perfect meal, shared with those we love, preferably whilst lazing under a leafy shade on a warm summer's day. Food is traditionally the way the matriarch of the family feeds us, making us feel loved and cherished. Some of our happiest memories are meals shared with family and friends; adults laughing and children playing around a table laden with our favorite foods. The very thought can stimulate those feeling-good emotions.

The current understanding about the happiness/food connection starts with the "emotional chemicals" and how they affect the brain. The very act of eating food gives us the right brain chemicals that make us feel warm and satisfied. These chemicals are called neurotransmitters. Their function is to send messages from one nerve cell to another within the brain and they influence thought, functions and feelings. Neurotransmitters are made in the brain from the food we eat and are highly sensitive to the type of foods that are eaten. In fact, they get all their nutrients from the food we eat, so if we don't eat the right foods, our brain can't help but underperform.

The neurotransmitters that are most sensitive to diet and most influential in affecting how we feel are **serotonin**, **dopamine** and **noradrenalin**.

THE EMOTIONAL CHEMICALS

Serotonin – the happy chemical

Serotonin is the most important chemical in terms of feeling good and can only be made by the brain. Foods rich in the amino acid tryptophan help the brain to make supplies of serotonin. Serotonin is associated with lifting the mood, decreasing feelings of stress and tension and helping us to relax. At night the brain converts serotonin into melatonin, which helps keep your internal clock on form and give you a good night's sleep.

Great serotonin-boosting foods are: bananas, turkey, cottage cheese, sunflower seeds, brown rice, peanuts and soy products.

Dopamine – the pleasure pursuit chemical

Dopamine is a neurotransmitter whose function is to get you to pursue things that give you pleasure, like eating, sex and feeling loved and cherished. It helps keep your brain alert, aids concentration, short-term memory and clarity of thinking. It is also necessary for producing noradrenalin (see below). Like serotonin, dopamine is made by the brain by converting an amino acids into the neurotransmitter, and the foods that specifically do that are rich in tyrosine. The very act of eating triggers a release of dopamine that gives a pleasure feeling, so it's important to moderate the production of dopamine to avoid overeating and becoming obese. Dopamine works best when you need a mood boost or you are stressed out and need a little lift to help you get over a tricky patch.

Great tyrosine foods are: lean chicken, fresh fish, cottage cheese, sunflower seeds, dried beans and bananas.

Noradrenalin – the stress-busting chemical

The noradrenalin neurotransmitter is for helping with stress and fear, and keeping your brain alert, enabling you to feel more motivated, attentive and more mentally energetic. It is made from dopamine, which comes from foods rich in tyrosine. The levels of noradrenalin can affect your mood, with too little leading to depression and tiredness, whilst too much can leave you feeling anxious. When noradrenalin is released into the bloodstream it acts like a hormone and has the effect of raising blood pressure and heart rate; it is vital in the "fight or flight" reaction that occurs in times of stress.

Great tyrosine foods are listed above.

These emotional chemicals are the starting point for eating foods that fight depression. But, taking our diet as a whole, we want to include whole grains to help balance our blood-sugar levels and avoid the "sugar low," fresh vegetables for their cleansing properties which will help us feel lighter, fresh fruit for their amazing enzymes and antioxidants which protect us, and beans and pulses for their energy force. These and other vital foods that help fight depression are explained throughout the book; turn to Chapter 5 to find out more about the superfoods to fight depression.

IS YOUR DIET STRESSING YOU OUT?

Of course, it's not just what you're leaving out that affects how you feel; it's also what you are putting in that affects how stressed, tired or depressed you are. The more you eat the high-fat, high-salt, high-sugar foods that have become the norm in our modern diet, the less happy you will feel. This is extensively covered in Chapter 4 ("Bad-Mood Foods") but suffice to say that if you do feel depressed, it could be more to do with your diet than you think.

According to a paper published in February 2005 by the US Department of Agriculture, Economic Research Service, 75 percent of the world's food is "processed" in some way. Processed foods are foods not in their natural state, and many of these foods are high in saturated fats, sugar and salt, which are detrimental to our emotional health. In fact, if you look at what most people have in their supermarket trolleys, you will see that it is unusual for anyone to have no processed or junk food and, as a society, we have come to consider processed foods as "normal."

This can create a vicious cycle:

We eat to change the way we feel
The processed food we eat gives us cravings
We eat to satisfy the cravings
We feel lousy and, to compensate, we eat more processed food
We then feel more awful
And we eat to change the way we feel

When you are hungry and you rush into the supermarket to buy something for dinner, the processed foods look like the perfect, quick answer to a busy schedule. Grabbing a "ready meal" can seem the utopia for any of us whose lives don't accommodate the pleasure of cooking at home. My friend Fiona sums it up with her comment, "If I can't get it from my local supermarket and cook it in five minutes, I'm not interested!" However, these types of foods have a knock-on effect and can leave us feeling emotionally drained and debilitated.

Depression is not an isolated state of emotional misery. When we become depressed we can also feel stressed and fatigued. The three are inextricably linked. If we are depressed we may go for the type of food that will give us "comfort," like alcohol, caffeine, cakes and cookies, chocolate or a fat-filled treat like pizza or fries.

These foods will give us a shot of mood-altering endomorphine-type substances which make us feel "high" or which temporarily numb our feelings. However, the downside to these foods is the drop in energy and good-mood levels which takes place afterwards and may result in us feeling worse than before we started. We then experience fatigue and anxiety, which results in us feeling bad about ourselves and, worse, can render us feeling even more depressed. Again, it's a vicious cycle.

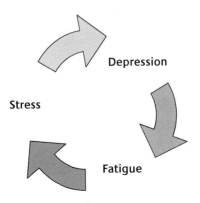

Depression

Stress

Fatigue

Depression has soared in the last few decades and the World Health Organization believes that we will be at an epidemic stage by 2020. At the same time, the production and sales of processed foods have also soared. According to a food survey carried out by the US Department of Agriculture, the purchase of processed foods over the last 25 years has significantly increased, and a food survey carried out by the UK Department for Environment, Food and Rural Affairs (DEFRA), confirms this. Here are some samples from their most recent figures.

Foodstuff	Percentage change in purchasing per person from 1975–2000
Dairy desserts	+ 6500%
Processed cheese	+50%
Processed vegetables (tinned, frozen)	+37%
Crisps and potato snacks	+225%
Frozen desserts	+350%
Vegetable ready meals	+5600%
Processed meat products (sausages, pies, etc)	+24%
Yogurt and fromage frais	+388%

The huge rise in processed desserts accounts for much of the large amount of sugar that we eat and sugar is top of the list of bad-mood foods. We buy more ready meals than ever before, including vegetable ready meals; this may indicate how we purchase processed vegetables as opposed to buying fresh vegetables. We are also buying more quick snack foods, which come with a high salt content. Information on soft drinks has only been available sine 1992, but since then our purchase and consumption has risen by 38%.

Here we have the purchasing figures for the four main staples of a good-mood food diet:

Foodstuff	Percentage change in purchasing per person from 1975–2000
Fresh green vegetables	-32%
Dried pulses (beans, peas, etc.)	-67%
Fresh potatoes	-45%
Flour	-57%

We are buying much less fresh vegetables. This may leave us vulnerable to buying a "quick meal" from the supermarket. Potatoes are purchased less frequently but we are buying more processed potato foods like frozen fries. Dried pulses are on the decrease and these are an excellent food for helping to beat depression and fatigue as they are high in fiber, protein and have a low Glycemic Index (GI). The decrease in flour purchasing means that we are baking less and relying more on ready-baked foods like cakes, bread and pastries to supplement our diets; the problem with these foods is they are high in salt, sugar and trans fats, all of which contribute to a low mood. If we bake ourselves we have more control over our ingredients.

FOOD FOR THOUGHT

It's often said that we had a great diet during World War II. We were much healthier because many of our favorite foods were restricted by the government.

Although everyone complained about the lack of variety in the wartime diet, there were tremendous health benefits because children who grew up during the period ate low-fat, low-sugar and high-fiber foods. After the war was over, manufacturing of processed foods went into full swing, delighting the population with highly flavored foods. In fact, canned and frozen foods were seen as a luxury that everyone could afford. My grandmother still remembers the way that processed food was the ultimate luxury and one-upmanship rivalry took place over who had the most canned and frozen foods in their house.

It's not just our diet that has changed; our way of eating has also altered. We have moved from the "three square meals a day" to a new precedent. Fifty years ago offices, factories and shops would close in the middle of the day to allow everybody to go home and eat a home-cooked lunch. But now we either grab what we can off the supermarket shelf and eat it on the go, or buy convenience food and ready meals that are heated up in a microwave. Our overall diet has changed from unrefined, low-fat, fiber-rich, plant-based foods to a highly processed, snack-focused, intensively farmed diet—the types of food that I believe are proving to make us depressed.

On the one hand we've never had it so good, with a fabulous array of international cuisine readily available in local restaurants, takeaways and home-delivery outlets. But on the other hand, ready-made and processed foods are fast becoming a real dilemma because of their high fat, salt and sugar content. The statistics deliver the evidence that the more processed food we eat, the poorer our general health is becoming and the more depression we are suffering.

The way the family eats is also changing. Family mealtimes are becoming so rare that one in four homes no longer has a dinner table for people to sit round. If families want to eat together, more and more they have to sit next to one another on the couch. Couch meals are more likely to be made up of processed foods or TV dinners rather than a home-cooked meal. This is backed up by a study from Tufts University in Boston where a lead researcher states, "High television viewing goes along with a cluster of family food behaviors where people tend to be unfocused. They want easy routines, no muss, no fuss. When a family is in that kind of mode there is a tendency to reach for easy solutions and that is processed foods."

> We rarely sit down as a family to eat because our lifestyle doesn't allow it. I come in late from work and get a quick meal on for the kids. They eat it in front of the TV while I change because I usually have a work commitment. My husband will cater for himself while I grab a mouthful of the leftovers as I'm grabbing my keys. I know it's not right but I'm too busy and too stressed to change it!
> JENNA KILLNER, AGED 44

MIXED MESSAGES

In spite of all the information that is available to us, it is sometimes hard to siphon off what really counts and what doesn't. The sheer volume of information can leave us feeling impotent in our decision-making process. The statistics are also frightening and are leading us toward a modern neurosis about food. There is a new term for people taking healthy-eating plans to an extreme: "orthorexia." This is driving people to become as obsessively compulsive about eating healthily as people with severe eating disorders. We receive mixed messages from the huge barrage of information we receive from all forms of media:

✳ Statements about how much longer we are living compared to previous generations, yet we have a one in four chance of dying of cancer.
✳ We are shown pictures of perfectly slim people looking sexy and beautiful as they eat their chocolate bars, but we know if we eat those same bars, we won't look like that.
✳ We are told that we are not taking in enough nutrients from food and we need supplements but then we discover that some supplements may be a danger to our health.

❋ We read that in order to feel good we need to clear out our food cupboards and take extreme measures with eating plans, but other gurus tell us that "normal" eating is the way to good emotional health – the term "normal" is ambiguous and confusing.

We have to make decisions in the face of too many conflicting arguments and can become dizzy with the onslaught of such information.

For many people food is not so much the basis for self-nourishment as a source of anguish, guilt and shame. Branded processed food has become a huge money-spinner so that celebrities are paid to encourage us and our children to eat foods that are damaging to our health. But then again, we have a feast of reality TV programs telling us how unhealthy we are, and how we have to change everything we eat in order to stay healthy.

UNDERSTANDING WHAT THE BODY NEEDS

A simple understanding of what we need comes from the principle that our bodies require protein, carbohydrates, vitamins, minerals, fats and water every day (in varying amounts depending on our sex, weight etc.) in order to stay well. The body must have these nutrients. But if we don't feed ourselves with a balanced diet then our bodies must get these nutrients from our organs—which are where our internal nutritional stores sit. If our bodies have to feed off our organs for too long we will begin to feel bad, become stressed, suffer fatigue and develop headaches.

Your body needs food to maintain energy, growth and repair, and to function properly and fight off stress and depression. A regular diet, including a high proportion of whole-grain products, fruit and vegetables and a low proportion of fat and sugars, will provide your body with good nutrition and high energy levels.

These are the nutrients your body needs.

Carbohydrates

Carbohydrates are broken down into glucose, which is either used as energy or stored as glycogen in the liver and muscles. The best carbohydrates for your body are those with a low Glycemic Index (GI). These are slow-burning foods that produce a steady level of sugar into the bloodstream, which will give you prolonged energy rather than a feeling of tiredness. To fight depression you should eat low-GI foods, like low-fat protein foods (nuts, beans and lentils), whole grains, fruit and vegetables, which will provide plenty of slow-release energy. Food producers are starting to put the GI of a food on packaging for easy recognition.

Protein

Protein is used to build and repair cells and is provided by foods such as beans, pulses, poultry, nuts, seeds, meat, fish and soya. Too little protein can cause loss of lean tissue, which may leave you feeling tired and prone to fatigue—this can lead to depression.

Healthy fats

Your body needs some essential fatty acids, and particularly omega-3, for boosting your mood.

Vitamins and minerals

The many different vitamins and minerals help your body to stay healthy, function properly and to fight disease and depression. Fruit and vegetables are good sources of vitamins and minerals.

Fiber

Your body does not absorb fiber, but it helps to keep the digestive system healthy. When your digestive system is healthy you may feel "lighter" and less sluggish, with more energy. Fiber is found in fruit and vegetables, whole-grain bread and cereals, as well as beans, lentils, nuts and seeds.

A quick glance at this food chart will give you an overall idea of the volumes of foods you should eat to gain the nutrients your body needs:

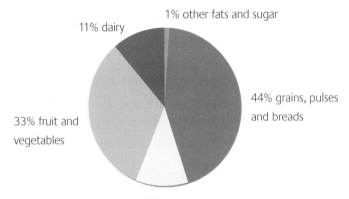

1% other fats and sugar

11% dairy

44% grains, pulses and breads

33% fruit and vegetables

11% meat

UNDERSTANDING WHAT EMOTIONS NEED

Knowing our emotions and having an awareness of the way we feel can become our guide in assessing how well we are eating. If we are lacking in one area—let's say, for example, we feel tired, which may lead to depression—we can find some "good energy food" and include it in our food plan for a few days until we feel more energetic. Observing how we feel is an excellent indicator of how well we are eating. By incorporating some ideas for good-mood food we can become our own best food guru.

One of the huge benefits that comes from changing the way we eat and incorporating fresher—and less-processed—foods into our diet is that not only do we feel more energetic but we feel cleaner! It's true: once you start eating good-mood food, you get a different sensation of your body and what it needs. You find that cravings for high-sugar, fatty and salty foods decrease. You may also start to feel less depressed and more positive as a result of feeling cleaner; it works inside and out.

When you start to feel physically fitter and emotionally buoyant, your body gets to know that feeling—it doesn't want to go back to feeling sluggish after it has had some experience of feeling energized, alive and strong. A natural inclination toward energizing, mood-boosting foods will creep into your intention without you even recognizing it. After following one of the 7-Day Food Plans you may become more aware of how your diet affects the way you feel. This is one of the most empowering discoveries, because it puts you right in charge of your wellbeing.

In the same way as implementing a long-term exercise plan—rather than a five-day mad dash to the gym—a leaning toward good food for better long-term health is of far greater benefit than extreme dietary changes. We can compound new eating ideas by attending to our relationship with our bodies and becoming more aware of how certain foods affect our emotions. We can learn to support our emotions through nourishing our bodies, and can gradually become comfortable with these two parts of ourselves, learning to bring them together through a change in how we eat.

IS YOUR DIET AFFECTING YOUR MOOD?

If you are unclear whether or not your food is affecting the way you feel, then here is a simple questionnaire that will help you establish just how much your diet may be contributing to your emotional wellbeing. Score yourself in the boxes on the right and see the results below.

Question	Every day – 3 points 2/3 times a week – 2 points Rarely – 1 point Never – 0 points
Do you eat more than one high-sugar snack, e.g. piece of cake or a couple of cookies?	
Do you have more than one unit of alcohol, e.g. a glass of wine?	
Do you eat less than 2 portions of fresh vegetables?	
Do you feel tired after you have eaten a meal?	
Do you drink less than 2 glasses of water?	
Do you rely on convenience foods for your main meals?	
Do you eat in front of the television?	
Do you suffer from headaches after eating?	
Do you grab some snack food when you are hungry, e.g. a bar of chocolate?	
How often do you go without a piece of fresh fruit?	
How often do you eat fried foods, e.g. fries?	
Do you feel bloated after eating a meal?	
Do you ever feel depressed about the food you eat?	
Do you keep breaking promises to yourself about eating better?	
Do you ever miss breakfast?	
How often do you go through the day on snacks rather than 3 meals a day?	
Do you feel depressed after eating?	
How often do you skip main meals?	
Do you eat high-salt foods, e.g. a bag of chips/nuts?	
How often do you eat takeaway meals, e.g. pizza, Chinese, curry?	
TOTAL	

Scoring:

1–20: Your eating habits are generally healthy; it is unlikely that your diet is depressing your mood. You are not allowing too much processed food into your diet. If you are depressed it may be more to do with a trauma that is unresolved—see "Life Changes That Affect Mood" in Chapter 2.

21–40: Your diet is probably contributing to your depression. You may have erratic eating habits, which could exacerbate stress. When you get stressed you may find yourself relying on quick-energy foods with a high GI factor, which means they are digested quickly and this leaves you feeling hungry more often. Your balance of foods may be out of kilter if you are relying on snacks to see you through the day rather than wholesome fresh meals, and this can be contributing to fatigue, lethargy and depression.

41–60: Your diet is unbalanced, which means that you are probably eating high amounts of salt, sugar and saturated fats in your diet—these can definitely contribute to depression. If you feel depressed you may find yourself turning to snacks and processed foods for comfort and these kind of foods can create a "numbing out" effect and cause you to lose mental focus and clarity (see "Bad-Mood Foods" in Chapter 4). Once you find yourself in this vicious cycle, your craving for highly processed foods becomes strong and it can be hard to break the habit. There is a high probability that changing your food will change your mood.

The good news

The great news is you can change your eating habits and change the way you feel. If you want a simple food plan to get you going, go straight to the three 7-Day Food Plans which start on page 169 and there you will find simple and fun food plans to get you started on feeling happy, calm and energized!

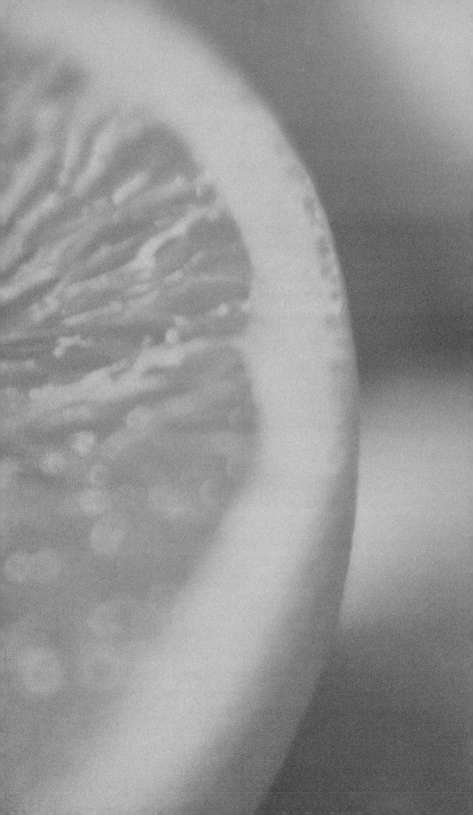

2
EATING TO BEAT DEPRESSION

Can it be true? Can we really eat our way to beating depression? If you are severely depressed it can feel like you're in the middle of a powerful whirlpool that is dragging you down and, in spite of your very best efforts, you just can't grab onto anything to get a grip. And, as the water engulfs you and the strength of the whirlpool pulls you under, you might not feel there is any way out. Well, there is.

> When I was really depressed I ate chocolates, cheese and ice cream. They had a sort of zone-out effect on me. I went into a bit of a comatose state which, looking back, didn't help me at all, but at the time I never questioned whether what I was eating may have made me feel like that. I liked it—for an hour or two, but then I would feel sick and bad and I hated myself, which made me carry on eating that type of stuff in a sort of punishment. Since cleaning up my diet, I feel 150 percent better and I don't crave those types of food anymore but, if I do have a blowout, I feel depressed and down the next day and usually end up crying. I can't understand why the doctor didn't ask me about my diet. All he said was I had bipolar disorder and would probably need to go on drug treatment for the rest of my life! I never took the pills but just changed my food instead, which helped me to tackle my other problems.
>
> GINNY HUME, AGED 33

Here are some general guidelines that you can follow which will help you straighten out your eating habits and get you on the road to beating depression with a great diet.

FIVE A DAY

One recommendation for nourishing our bodies to boost our mood is to implement the "five-a-day" rule.

THINK COLOR: Here's a chart to get you thinking about the "Five a Day" color in your diet

Tomatoes. Peppers. Strawberries. Cranberries

Carrots. Oranges. Mango. Peaches. Pumpkin

Bananas. Sweetcorn. Nuts. Garbanzo beans

Broccoli. Avocado. Kale. Peppers. Beans

Blueberries. Eggplant. Blackberries. Raisins

Onions. Oats. Cauliflower. Garlic. Almonds

Scientific studies from the World Health Organization, the US Food and Drug Administration, the UK Department of Health, as well as many others, recommend eating a minimum of five portions of fruit and vegetables a day. Fruit and vegetables help to protect us from illnesses that take time to develop. What we eat now will affect our health in twenty years' time—the time taken for some illnesses, such as heart disease and cancer, to develop.

It's a double-edged sword: our immune system is lowered by chronic stress, which is a symptom of depression—but continued suppression of the immune system can lead to illness. People who are ill are therefore more likely to feel lethargic and debilitated—and lethargy and debilitation can lead to depression.

By way of contrast, happy people make for healthy people. One study has shown that feeling good reduces the risk of disease. "There's a direct link between how we're feeling and the biological processes which relate to illness and illness risk," said study author Dr. Andrew Steptoe, the British Heart Foundation Professor of Psychology at University College London. "Biology is going to be on the side of those people who are going to be in a more positive state of mind, and it may well stand these people in good stead for their future health."

By making sure we keep ourselves healthier, we are helping ourselves stay happier. In fact, the evidence shows that eating at least five portions of fruit and vegetables each day has very real health benefits—it could help prevent up to 20 percent of deaths from our nation's biggest killers—heart disease and some cancers.

Here are some examples of how Five a Day help you maintain good health:

* Vitamin A is essential for growth and the normal function of the retina of the eye. Red, orange and yellow fruits and vegetables are a good source.
* Vitamin E, found in vegetable oils, seed oils, cereals and avocado pears, is a potent antioxidant, involved in the formation of body tissues.
* Fruits and vegetables are sources of a range of antioxidants, the so-called ACE vitamins (vitamins A, C and E), which help to prevent DNA damage.
* Lycopene, found in tomatoes, and the compound lutein, found in broccoli, spinach and red peppers, are also potent antioxidants.
* Sinigrin, from Brussels sprouts, helps to protect us from cancer. It works by persuading pre-cancerous cells to commit suicide by a natural process called apoptosis.
* Sulphoraphane, from broccoli, also has powerful anti-cancer effects but, unlike sinigrin, it works by blocking cancer rather than suppressing it.
* Vitamin K, found in fresh green vegetables and fruit, is necessary for normal blood clotting.
* Vitamin B is made up of several compounds essential for a healthy metabolism. Green leafy vegetables, mushrooms and fruit are good sources.

The beneficial components of fruit and vegetables reinforce one another, and of course we get the best overall effect by eating a wide range of produce.

Just by implementing the "Five-a-Day" rule you can begin to change elements of your diet. For example, by adding more vegetables into a main meal, not only do you have less room for processed foods, but you will have less taste for processed foods. Your palate will change and you will have less of a craving for high-fat, high-salt and sugary foods. It's a great feeling going to sleep feeling satisfied but light because of a good-mood food dinner; or, going to work feeling sated with goodness and composure but energized because of a good-mood food breakfast.

To simplify the "Five-a-Day" rule, a portion is more or less what you can fit into your hand.

Here is a guide to what can be included in a "Five a Day" list:

✳ 1 apple, banana, pear, orange or other similar-sized fruit
✳ 2 plums or similar-sized fruit
✳ Half a grapefruit or avocado
✳ 1 slice of large fruit, such as melon or pineapple
✳ 3 heaped tablespoons of vegetables (raw, cooked, frozen or tinned)
✳ 3 heaped tablespoons of beans and pulses (however much you eat, beans and pulses count as a maximum of one portion a day)
✳ 3 heaped tablespoons of fruit salad (fresh or tinned in fruit juice) or stewed fruit
✳ 1 heaped tablespoon of dried fruit (such as raisins and apricots)
✳ 1 cupful of grapes, cherries or berries
✳ a dessert bowl of salad
✳ a glass (150ml) of fruit juice (however much you drink, fruit juice counts as a maximum of one portion a day)

It seems a simple task to follow the "Five-a-Day" rule, yet the average person eats only three portions a day. However, although it may seem hard to commit yourself to "Five a Day," here are some easy ways to accomplish the goal.

Keep stocks of fruit and vegetables at home

When you open the refrigerator to an eyeful of apples, pears, grapes and oranges, together with some fresh broccoli, a plump cauliflower, a bunch of carrots and some wholesome cabbage, it sets the scene for better eating. As obvious as it may sound, having the produce in your kitchen is one good way of helping yourself to get your "five a day."

Snack foods

When you need to stave off hunger pangs, resist the chocolate temptation and go for something fruity instead. At home, make sure that there is a fruit bowl everyone can see. This helps to bypass the potato chips, sodas and high-sugar snacks. Send children out with a bag of peeled and chopped carrots rather than a cereal bar. Carry an apple in your bag for a "just in case" moment. Buy some dried fruits instead of candy and add them to unsalted nuts.

Add to your cooking

Add sliced zucchini to your spaghetti bolognaise, roast apples to your Sunday roast pork, sliced peppers to your macaroni cheese and some sautéed mushrooms and grilled tomatoes to your breakfast. For dessert, make an apple pie, strawberries and cream, and real fruit Jell-O for the children.

Choose meals that are packed with veggies

If you are having soup for a dinner, you can add plenty of vegetables. If pasta is on the menu, remember that tomato-based spaghetti sauce counts as a vegetable. Having frozen pizza for a weekend lunch? Buy a plain one and add mushrooms, leeks, red and green peppers and onions.

Make a fruit salad

A home-made fruit salad is simple and can take ten minutes to prepare. You can chop fruit and then add a can of fruit in its own juice; this will give it some liquid and stop your apples going brown. Alternatively, buy a pack of mixed dried fruit from your local health store and soak in water overnight. A fruit salad makes a great breakfast, a snack for when you get in from work and you're starving, and a great dessert. It can last up to three days and you can use all seasonal fruit. For the good-mood benefit, eat some cornflakes for one breakfast and then eat a fruit salad the next day. Notice how good you feel after eating the fruit salad. And one portion of fruit salad can count as two portions of fruit and vegetables.

Drink up

Either choose 100 percent fruit and vegetable juices or juice your own—an easy and delicious way to add healthy produce to your diet.

For quick fixes, try one of these:

- **Munch** an apple after breakfast to feel *'cleaner'*
- **Cut up** some carrots, celery or other favorite foods and dip them into a tomato salsa (bought or home-made) to feel *more energy*
- **Blend** one kiwi fruit and one glass of juice (per person) to give you a shot of enzymes that will give you an *immediate lift*
- **Have a few** dried apricots, figs or dates to *placate hunger*
- **Eat** a banana to help *combat stress*

THREE MEALS A DAY

When we're depressed, overstressed or suffering from chronic fatigue, grazing through the day can become a habit which encourages us to eat the high-fat/salt/sugar foods as a comfort, in order to get the sugar high or simply because we have lost the habit of regularity in our life and in our food. Adopting the "Three Meals a Day" habit is a great way to bring back some stability, consistency and good order, which will spread into every other part of our daily routine.

The Three Meals a Day plan means just that: eating three good, fulfilling, nutritious meals that will help us with many areas. If we follow a food plan, like the ones outlined in Chapter 6, we will begin to bring some balance into our diet. It is a nurturing way to honor our body and state of mind, and the practice of thinking ahead to plan our meals is a way of taking good care of our emotional wellbeing.

> When I was at my rock bottom of a hellhole and my life was falling apart, I paid no attention to what I was eating and I ate as and when ... I felt like a child, out of control, and this spilled out into other ways I behaved—or the chaos I experienced meant I ate randomly, I don't know which came first. I heard someone talking about eating three meals a day and nothing in between and I thought it seemed so rigid and hard, but I began to adopt this idea. I noticed that after a couple of days I began to feel steadier and, though it was hard to give up the snacks, I did start to turn the corner. I felt physically better and got other stuff more under control. I'm not rigid about it but I do like orderly eating now and I do feel better about myself.
>
> Paul Warham, aged 39

With Three Meals a Day we are making a commitment to ourselves to stop snacking and this is powerful in itself, because when we snack we generally don't run for the carrot sticks and houmous but tend to dive into chips, cakes and cookies etc., which have no benefit to us except to make us feel worse. If you are hungry between meals then the snacks to be found in Chapter 6 will help sustain you to the next meal and have the added bonus of giving you some extra nutrients that processed foods wouldn't contain. It's a tricky one because sometimes we are looking for extra snacks because we are craving certain food such as sugar and salt, but in eating three substantial meals a day, we can find that these cravings quickly diminish.

In eating three good meals a day we also gain the benefit of a better balance in our sugar levels. Starting with a large breakfast (particularly good are oats or other low-GI foods) will give you a steady release of energy that might see you through to lunch. Then eating a lunch with a protein that contains tyrosine will help keep you alert for the afternoon. A dinner with tryptophan will help you to calm down and your body will produce melatonin, which will help you sleep. It is so exciting to recognize that you might be able to better regulate how you feel by a good eating plan and feel the benefits within 24 hours.

EXERCISE YOUR MIND

Working up a sweat might be just the thing for supporting your Emotional Eating recovery. A report from the Chartered Society of Physiotherapy goes as far to say that exercise is the *best* form of therapy for depression, with 57 percent of respondents stating that exercise has lifted their depression.

Exercise also reduces anxiety, gives you energy and floods the body with endorphins—the pleasure-inducing hormones that make you feel great. But this doesn't mean you need to work up a sweat in the gym; simply getting moving is enough to feel the benefits.

Walking is the best all-round exercise and you can adapt it for your own level of fitness. For the extremely unfit, just start walking instead of taking transport. Walk up and down stairs instead of taking the elevator. Or, take a walk when you feel like Emotional Eating. As you walk, don't go beyond a slightly increased breathing rate but build up your strength each time so that you can gain extra fitness from your walks.

When you walk you see the world from a different perspective. You become more in tune with your surroundings and community. Walking with animals or children can inspire your soul and give you a mental lift. If neither of these is available to you, you could offer your help at local clubs that need adults to accompany children in outdoor activities.

Gardening is a lovely way to boost the mood and the body. Being in touch with nature is a brilliant way to focus on pleasure, and the exercise required to mow, weed, dig and plant will stimulate both your brain and your heart. If you have no garden, help a neighbor out in their garden. Not only is this good exercise, it might lift you out of the loneliness that comes with depression.

Make exercise sociable by meeting up with friends and going on a joint bike ride. Picnics inspire outdoor games; take a ball and a bat or racket and propose a game of baseball, softball, football or tennis. The team game is a fun mood-lifter, with banter and support playing a nourishing part in lifting you out of the isolation of depression.

Swimming can be a form of meditation for some. Swimming lengths is an excellent workout but also provides the calming assurance of rhythm as you flow up and down the pool. Swimming is good for helping to fight stress and anxiety, as the effort required to get you through fifteen minutes of breaststroke leaves less to focus on what is wrong in your life and can help you to sleep better.

Dancing is springing up everywhere. Salsa, jive or ballroom dancing have become so fashionable that bars and clubs are lending themselves as dance halls for a couple of nights a week. The age groups span all generations, leaving less room for someone who is depressed to compare themselves with everyone else. The workout from the dancing can be intense if you join in every dance and that, combined with the friendliness of most people, means you can leave a class feeling really, really good.

You may find that the fitter you feel the better you feel. You also have a tool to keep your weight down. These two things are powerful in helping to fight depression as so many people, particularly women, feel depressed because of their weight. If you include some exercises to help you become more flexible, you may feel the benefits and pleasure that comes from being able to move better around your body. It is good to be able to pick something up without stiffness or pain and this can act as a great emotional boost as you may feel less physically and emotionally "stuck." Yoga is a great way to increase flexibility as well as decrease stress. A study from the Center for Integrative Medicine at Thomas Jefferson University, Philadelphia in 2003 found that yoga can be a form of moderate exercise that can help anyone to feel just a little better because it elicits a decrease in the levels of the stress hormone cortisol, which can lead to a greater sense of wellbeing.

How much should you do?

Your doctor is the best judge of that and can help determine the best exercise routine for you. You may consider some key factors, such as your age, sex, weight and goals. For a general guide, here are some ideas:

✷ Exercise at least three times a week for thirty minutes
✷ As you get fitter, increase your goals
✷ Make it fun or you won't stick with it
✷ Go outside as much as you can; the sun will increase your Vitamin D, which helps to lift the mood
✷ Drink lots of water – dehydration can leads to fatigue and therefore depression
✷ Whatever your age, exercise can help your depression

When we are depressed and turn to Emotional Eating for support, exercise can seem like a drag. The irony is that exercise will help curb Emotional Eating, because you will

receive a physical lift which may be enough to tip you into a
different state of mind, for example, "I feel a little better so I
won't eat the pizza I had in mind; I'll go for the stir-fry instead."
If you only do this once you will feel the benefit and your mind
will remember the experience. Exercise won't cure depression
but then there isn't one cure; there are several approaches to
beating depression of which exercise is one.

PREPARE – PREPARE – PREPARE

OK, you're following one of the 7-Day Plans, but you find
yourself stuck somewhere where you can't get to a selection of
fresh fruit and vegetables and you're starving. What do you do?
Buy the easiest thing to eat: a bag of chips, a pre-packed
sandwich or a cake. It can also be the case where you get
home and open the refrigerator but there's nothing there and
so you grab what you can, or call for a takeaway—and it's not
going to be the wholesome, complex-carbohydrate, rich in
enzymes, brimming with omega-3, depression-busting meal!
No, it's more likely to be the fat/sugar/salt-laden food that offers
a helping of fatigue, depression and diet stress!

The solution is to be prepared. This means thinking about
the food that you are going to eat tomorrow—today. By being
one step ahead of your hunger you will start to change lifetime
habits of grabbing whatever's going. Foods that fight depression
need a little planning and it can mean the difference between
feeling down in the dumps or on top of the world. Here are
ten tips to help you be prepared.

✱ Make a note of what you will eat tomorrow; this will give
  you time to check your recipes, even pore over a book and
  savor the thought of a new recipe that you're going to try,
  and jot down what ingredients you will need to organize to
  ensure you have all the components to hand.

✳ Do this after you have eaten and you will be more measured about what you decide to eat tomorrow.

✳ If you need to go shopping, make a list of what you need to buy and decide which shop you will use.

✳ Keep lists simple and make it as uncomplicated as possible because you want to ease yourself in gently when making these changes; don't put yourself off by making it awkward for you to get started.

✳ By following one of the 7-Day Food Plans you have all the preparation done for you, but remember to put aside time to get any specialized foods—like aduki beans, for instance—from a health shop.

✳ Remember to do your preparation the night before, e.g., if you need to soak beans or precook some rice.

✳ If you work away from home and you will be taking food with you for lunch, make sure you have this prepared or at least organized the night before to prevent the morning rush in which you might abandon the whole idea of taking in food to work and decide to grab some processed food at the last minute.

✳ Make time in your day to cook your main meal. For instance, when you come back from work, instead of slumping in front of the telly with a cup of coffee and a biscuit, get going on the supper straight away.

✳ If you always come home starving, prepare yourself by having good-mood foods in the house that you can sink your teeth into, e.g. a handful of toasted mixed nuts and seeds, oat cookies and peanut butter, wholewheat bread and honey, fresh fruit salad, a handful of home-made muesli (all recipes can be found in Chapter 6).

✳ With this book you can become canny at preparing your day's food around how you want to feel; if you want energy you can eat some protein like garbanzo beans, if you want to sleep well you can eat some carbohydrates like wholewheat pasta—how incredible is that!

THE GREAT DROUGHT

Did you know that we can often mistake thirst for hunger? We may be dehydrated and we don't realize it. Have you ever had a time when you were really thirsty but had no water to hand? You may have found that by the time you have got to a tap, your thirst had gone. This is the body adapting to dehydration, and means you may have lost the ability to recognize thirst. The reason that we need to drink lots of water is because dehydration causes fatigue, which can lead to depression.

One of the reasons we feel better in summer is because we drink more. The body loses up to two liters of water a day through normal bodily functions and this is the amount we need to drink to ensure we have all the benefits of hydration. If we are consuming enough water our organs will be nourished, our digestive system will function better, aches and pains may become less painful and our concentration span will increase. The brain is 85 percent water and a glass of water may be all it takes to feel a little better when you need a lift.

* Dry mouth
* Thirst
* Dry tongue
* Fuzzy head
* Lack of concentration
* Wrinkles
* Dark-coloured urine
* Depression
* Stress
* Fatigue
* Hangover

So to fight depression, make water a top priority. If you feel tired, try drinking one glass of water and you may be amazed just how much more energy you have.

BECOME A HAPPY SHOPPER

Are you a happy shopper? Or are you a "let's get the hell in and get the hell out again" shopper?

The supermarket spell

The supermarket assaults the senses but is difficult to avoid because it's where 80 percent of our grocery purchases happen. Before you arrive you are charmed with promises of discounted items and loyalty cards, but once you get there your wits are bombarded with millions of marketing dollars' worth of words and color, each trying to get you to buy that packet. The smells are powerful "Buy Me" tools: the roasted chickens, fresh pizzas, just-baked bread—but sometimes these are added smells designed to hook us in. Then choosing the food can be stressful with the overwhelming array of choice. And now we are being asked to question the labels on the packets, and very few people understand them!

But, finally, we go for the picture, because that Thai Green Chicken Curry with Almond and Cilantro Rice looks perfect for a little dinner for two with a bag of salad—the photo shows a sumptuous dish with all the right ingredients: not too much fat, rice (that's good) and lean chicken breast. But get it home and it is a disappointing green sludge of mess—on the other hand, it cost a whole lot of dollars and you're starving, so you wolf it down and vow not to buy it again. That is until the next time you go in, when all your vows of home cooking go out the window as you next fall in love with the picture on the cardboard wrapping with the words "deliciously authentic," "fresh ingredients" or "irresistible," all of which are allowed yet, legally, mean nothing.

The new trend is to have well-known chefs selling ready-prepared foods on the shelf with pictures of their faces on the products—but would top chefs use ingredients such as hydrogenated fats, dried glucose syrup, mono- and di-glycerides of fatty acids or acidity regulator in their restaurants? Probably not, but we eat them. Yet these can make us feel lethargic, sluggish and stressed, all of which are symptoms of depression.

Are you a happy shopper?

Tick each question with a 'yes' or 'no':

Question	Yes OR No
Do you get stressed as you walk into the supermarket?	
Do you find yourself lost for inspiration once inside?	
Do you go shopping without a list?	
Do you have no idea of a budget in mind?	
Do you ever go shopping when you're hungry?	
Do you go shopping without thinking of what you're going to cook with the food you're buying?	
Are you hypnotized by the packaging?	
Do you shop with children?	
Does the huge choice overwhelm you?	
Are you seduced by the photographs on the packets?	
Are you tempted to buy the bread or cakes when you smell the just-baked smell?	
Do you feel pressured by previous media advertising?	
Do you often spend over your budget?	
Are you seduced into buying things you didn't come in for, like CDs, make-up or a T-shirt?	
Are you tempted to buy something you can't afford because you are putting it on a credit card?	
Do you buy little treats that are not on your list?	
Do you buy snacks because you're hungry and eat them before you get to the till?	
Do you get fed up waiting in the queue at the deli?	
Do you grab a little something you don't need at the checkout queue – like a candy bar or chewing gum?	
Does your stress level rise when you're standing in the queue waiting to pay?	

If you have answered 'yes' eight or more times, you probably find the whole shopping experience to be stressful, frustrating or depressing. This quickly links to food and mood; by the time you've dragged your food home from the artificially lit supermarket, feeling slightly deranged after a twenty-minute fight to get through the till, you have lost the will to live let alone unpack the bags and cook the food. But there are other ways to make shopping a delicious experience that is a part of the whole ensemble of preparing food to fight depression.

Shopping online

This is a perfect stress-free way to shop! You can buy absolutely everything, including fresh vegetables and fruit, and the huge advantage is you can plan your weekly shopping easily, stick to the list and make sure you're not swayed by those tempting offers and impulse purchases. You can even see the packaging and get all the nutritional information you need—all from the comfort of your own home.

Farmers' markets

Farmers' markets are springing up everywhere; they are becoming the way that local producers can compete with the supermarket giants. When you go to a farmers' market you can be sure that the food sold is from a defined local area and the farmers, growers or producers are present in person to sell their own produce, direct to the public. All products sold should have been grown, reared, caught, brewed, pickled, baked, smoked or processed by the stallholder.

By wandering around the farmers' market you can ask questions about the food, how it's grown or made and what's in it. These markets are taking on the feel of the continental markets and they can be a delight—they remind me of being on vacation. To feel the food and get the growers' view on his produce is fun.

Street markets

Not as salubrious as a farmers' market, but street markets are a good source for good, cheap vegetables that cost less than those at the supermarket! Yes, less than the supermarket. We tend to think that the supermarket must be the cheapest because those adverts tell us with their marketing campaigns and "price cuts," but they are not cheaper for fresh produce.

One of the reasons we tend to think that markets are more expensive is that we buy our produce with cash. When we pay by credit card we tend to spend more but when we pay by cash it feels like we're spending a lot of money. In fact we're not, because we're not accruing interest payments as well.

Your local butcher, fishmonger or greengrocer

Go and check out your local butcher. He can tell you where the chicken has come from and what size you need for what meal; he will also offer a few tips for cooking: "Put a bunch of tarragon in the cavity before you roast it and it will taste superb." We just don't realize what a difference a local shop can make. If you're ill they may deliver; you can phone them to reserve you a sea bass; their shops exude a more continental style of shopping than the supermarkets. And again, you may find the prices to be less than your local supermarket.

Ten tips to becoming a happy supermarket shopper

However, if you *do* need to go into the supermarket for your regular shop, here are ten top tips for stress-free shopping:

* Never go in hungry because you will probably buy foods that you are craving because your blood-sugar level drops
* Always go in with a list and stick to it; this will make you feel so good because you will not be allowing the 'supermarket spin' to bias you
* Have a menu in mind before you go and relish buying the right foods, thereby nurturing your soul

* Be aware that certain smells might be there to seduce you and don't be tempted
* Don't take the kids
* Resist treats at the checkout – if you don't feel hungry you won't succumb
* Take your deli queue ticket and go and get some other products until your number is almost called – you will learn what speed shopping is all about
* Try to shop at a time when you are least depressed
* If you take cash you are better able to stick to your budget
* Remember the food chart, which will indicate how to, proportionately, fill your shopping basket (see page 22):

LIFE CHANGES THAT AFFECT MOOD

Of course, there may be some specific reasons why we are depressed that are not directly related to what we eat, although they could be exacerbated by a poor diet. There are certain life changes that happen which create stress—an all too familiar component of modern life. Not only are we trying to get through the day by dealing with traffic jams, busy shops and too little time, but we also have to manage life changes that can cause added stress and can lead to periods of prolonged depression. Yet when it comes to life stressors, do you know which life events are at the top of the suspect list?

Based on their famous 1967 studies, Dr. Thomas H Holmes and Dr. Richard H Rahe developed the Social Readjustment Rating Scale (SRRS). They had suggested that stressful events would be positively correlated with illness. The SRRS demonstrated a positive correlation between the total stress people experienced within a year and their increased chances of becoming ill, including depression. The following is a list of stress-inducing events, in the order of their Life Change Unit (LCU), from high to low.

Life Event	LCU
1. Death of spouse	100
2. Divorce	73
3. Marital Separation	65
4. Jail Term	63
5. Death of a close family member	63
6. Personal injury or illness	53
7. Marriage	50
8. Being sacked from work	47
9. Reconciliation with spouse	45
10. Retirement	45
11. Change in health of family member	44
12. Pregnancy	40
13. Sexual difficulties	39
14. Addition of family member	39
15. Major business readjustment	39
16. Major change in financial state	38
17. Death of a close friend	37
18. Changing to a different line of work	36
19. Change in frequency of arguments with spouse	35
20. Mortgage for loan or major purchase over £100,000	31
21. Foreclosure on a mortgage or loan	30
22. Major change in responsibilities at work	29
23. Children leaving home	29
24. Trouble with in-laws	29
25. Outstanding personal achievement	28
26. Spouse begins or stops work	26
27. Starting or ending school	26
28. Change in living conditions	25
29. Revision of personal habits (dress, manners, associations)	24
30. Trouble with boss	23
31. Change in work hours, conditions	20
32. Change in main residence	20
33. Change in school	20
34. Change in recreational activities	19
35. Change in church activities	19
36. Change in social activities	18
37. Mortgage or loan under £100,000	17
38. Change in sleeping habits	16

Life Event	LCU
39. Change in number of family gatherings	15
40. Change in eating habits	15
41. Holiday	13
42. Christmas	12
43. Minor violation of the law	11

Interestingly, not all stressful occasions are 'bad'. An Outstanding Personal Achievement is seen as a stressor even though it's a positive event. So, how many of the events in the list have you encountered in past twelve months? Identify them and add up their LCUs. Here is what Dr Holmes and Dr Rahe predict:

- Total LCU below 150: You have a 35% chance of illness or accident within the next two years
- Total LCU between 150 and 300: Your chance increases to 51%
- Total LCU over 300: Your chance increases to 80%

If your total LCU is high, it can be a great stress relief to know why. Using this survey you can begin to get a grip on the life changes that have brought you to this point where you may feel powerless over things that shape your life. By acknowledging the stress that these life changes have brought, you can begin to take action to make positive changes that can help to turn your life around. By also looking at your food and how this is contributing to your stressed state and depressed feelings, you can finally start to take a powerful step toward recovery.

3
EMOTIONAL
EATING

WHAT IS EMOTIONAL EATING?

We've all headed for the kitchen when we were upset and thought nothing of it. Having something to eat to appease a bad feeling is a way of life. What's more, we encourage it in others: "eat and you'll feel better," candy for the child who's fallen over, or a special meal to kiss and make up with your lover after a row. It's part of our culture and we are raised to believe that food represents something other than physical hunger. This is Emotional Eating—it's when we eat but we really want something else: approval, nurturing or to change bad feelings.

We're all Emotional Eaters, and why not? Who hasn't experienced feeling depressed and grabbing a candy bar to cheer themselves up? For some people, however, Emotional Eating isn't simply a quick "fix" for the blues; it is part of a continuous strategy to keep negative feelings away. The problem is the foods that change the way we feel are generally processed foods high in sugar, salt and saturated fats, all of which contribute to feeling bad. Continually turning to processed foods to manage feelings leads to cravings for more of the same, and so more depression sets in because of the negative effect of food and the original reasons for the depression.

This can lead to a chronic cycle of feeling bad, eating bad, feeling worse, eating more bad-mood food and feeling even worse ...

Feel numbed but physically worse, tired and depressed

Feel bad so eat to push feelings away

Need to eat processed foods to get a quick fix but brings self-hate

The cycle of Emotional Eating is a vicious one. We feel bad, we eat to "stuff down" the bad feelings, we feel ashamed of ourselves for stuffing our face, we feel guilty, our self-worth plummets, we eat junk food whilst thinking, "What the hell … what does it matter if I eat another pastry," so eat another one and feel wholly depressed. Once the cycle is in place the physical cravings come into play and you start longing for the junk foods and so the cycle continues.

According to research undertaken by the Priory Group in the UK, 43 percent of adults admitted that they eat to stifle negative feelings. The most common reasons for Emotional Eating are to suppress feelings of boredom, loneliness, stress or anger, or after arguing with a spouse or partner. Of the adults surveyed, 40 percent thought they were overweight, 25 percent thought they would be happier if they were thinner and 25 percent felt guilty after eating food.

We hear terms such as "eating disorder," "compulsive eating" or "food addiction," terms used to describe extreme eating patterns that are potentially very dangerous, but what about the millions of us who don't have these serious disorders but have simply got into the habit of turning to food when we feel things are getting on top of us and seem to have got into some bad habits? I have never met anyone who is depressed who doesn't turn to food in times of depression. But the biggest predicament is the type of food we turn to at these times—we don't turn to carrot sticks, healthy salads or fresh vegetables. Why not? Because these foods don't give us the "junk-food high" that chips, chocolate, fries, cookies and pizza can offer.

In July 2003, the *Sunday Times* printed an article entitled "Burgers Are As Addictive As Drugs" and discussed the argument that high doses of fat and sugar in processed foods can be as addictive as nicotine and even hard drugs. This is backed up by research undertaken in 2003 at the Rockefeller University, New York, which revealed that foods high in fat and sugar can cause significant changes in the brain's chemistry, with effects similar to powerful opiates such as morphine. This research states that regular eating of these foods can quickly reconfigure the body's hormonal system to want yet more fat. It can be a form of addiction; indeed, when alcoholics or addicts clean up they often have to attend to their fat/sugar/carb addiction because they gain copious amounts of weight which can threaten their health as much as the original addiction.

Double trouble

If you start to reap some of the penalties of this cycle of Emotional Eating, which can include physical illnesses like diabetes, heart disease and angina, you may be placed on drugs that often include other side effects like dizziness, feeling faint, breathlessness, sleepiness or insomnia. So, not only do you feel depressed, but the Emotional Eating cycle may have pointed you toward a whole new eating pattern, which can cause devastating diet-related diseases. The British Institute of Science in Society estimates that between 1995 and 2025, the number of adults affected by diabetes in developed countries will have increased by 41 percent. The American Diabetes Association says "studies show that people with diabetes have a greater risk of depression than people without diabetes."

At the same time your body could be reacting to the lack of good-mood boosters such as serotonin because of Emotional Eating. Foods with a high tryptophan count (that promote serotonin) such as lean chicken, fresh fish, cottage cheese, sunflower seeds, dried beans, or bananas might be excluded from your diet on a regular basis. The increased intake of sugar also creates an artificial "high" that may stop your brain from creating serotonin. This explains why people find it so difficult to stop turning to junk foods, because it takes the body some time to balance out its natural levels and get you feeling better.

The good news is that Emotional Eaters don't eat more than non-emotional eaters; the bad news is that they eat fats higher in fat/salt/sugar i.e. processed foods.

The problem is that when we feel depressed we can talk ourselves into justifying the first mouthful as a "comfort" or a "what the hell, I feel bad anyway and here's a little piece of enjoyment in my lousy day!" The eating action can produce feel-good endomorphines together with the sugar/carbohydrate rush and, hey presto: NO NEGATIVE EMOTIONS—IN FACT, NO EMOTIONS AT ALL!

ARE YOU AN EMOTIONAL EATER?

The good news is that there is a way to help you to begin to eat food without developing these destructive relationships. If you are depressed and you know it's really not because of your diet then please read my first book *Beat Depression and Reclaim Your Life*, which will help you through the devastation of depression and set you on your way to beating it. If you suffer from depression and you know you are an Emotional Eater then you can use the work plan in this book together with the work plan in *Beat Depression and Reclaim Your Life* and tackle your wellbeing on two fronts.

Before we begin here is a questionnaire to assess whether or not you are an Emotional Eater. Simply go through the questions and answer "yes" or "no" for each one:

Are you an emotional eater?	Yes/No
Do you eat when you feel depressed?	
If you feel depressed and eat to comfort yourself, is your depression temporarily lifted?	
Do you eat when you feel angry?	

Do you sometimes punish yourself after eating?

Do you sometimes feel numb after eating food?

Do you sometimes feel guilty after eating food?

Do you eat when you feel sad?

Does your weight fluctuate by more than 5lb in a 3-month period?

Do you feel under pressure to be thin?

Do you think about being thin as you eat?

Do you sometimes starve yourself as a punishment?

Do you eat when you feel lonely?

Do you turn to food or not eat enough when you are stressed?

Do you eat when you are bored?

Do you hide foods for you to eat later?

Do you turn to food or restrict your eating when you feel under pressure?

If you restrict yourself, do you feel more in control?

Do you fear losing control with your eating?

Do you sometimes eat and then feel a failure?

Do you smoke, exercise, or drink lots of caffeine to try and control your hunger?

Do you ever lie to others about what you have or haven't eaten?

Add up your "yes" answers. If you have scored eight or more, you are probably an Emotional Eater. This means that you sometimes eat food to compensate for how you are feeling and this might be when you are feeling bad. Being an Emotional Eater isn't necessarily obvious to anyone else, because it doesn't necessarily mean you are overweight, but you know that you use food to try and change the way you feel. The more "yes" answers you have scored the more pulling power food, particularly junk food, has on you. The more you feel you need to eat junk food to cope, the more depressed you may become.

WHAT TYPE OF EMOTIONAL EATER ARE YOU?

We all have a different favorite food we turn to in times of need and often this is food that children would eat: candy, chocolate, chips, cakes, etc. Dr. Christine Courbasson, Assistant Professor, Department of Psychiatry, University of Toronto, Canada, says that the urge to eat emotionally is instilled early in life. "Society has contributed to most people eating in response to their emotions. Children are given food when they are sad or as a reward when they behave well. We learn that this is acceptable, but in fact it is very dangerous."

The danger is in eating too much food, which can then cause health problems. But in identifying our own pattern of behavior we are better able to identify our eating patterns and that is the first step toward managing our Emotional Eating. Here are some common patterns of behavior. Decide which one you are; your choice of food can perhaps reveal your emotional needs.

Choice of food	Why	Emotional needs
Ice cream	Depressed	To be soothed
Salted nuts	Stressed	Take things more in your stride
Spiced foods	Restless/agitated	More spice in your life
Candy	Feel childlike	Self-talk from own internal adult side
Big portions	Unable to cope	More support
Creamy/cheesy foods	Lack of self-esteem	Some good feedback from peer group
Caffeine	Need energy	Physical exercise
Alcohol	Need to block out all emotions — maybe dealing with unresolved grief	Self-management

THE MOST COMMON REASONS FOR EMOTIONAL EATING

✻ Eating 'numb out' food defers dealing with pressures
✻ Emotional Eaters are caught up in the physical craving for sugary, fatty and salty foods
✻ Emotional Eaters are trying to fill a hungry heart
✻ Emotional Eaters haven't dealt with some historic loss

THE WEIGHTY ISSUE

If you've hit a bad patch and used Emotional Eating to cope with your feelings, you may have gained weight. Gaining weight is common with Emotional Eaters. As you turn to food to try and console yourself in hard times, it is hard to stick to the good-mood foods because you will probably be craving the high-fat/sugar/salt foods as these can "numb" the emotions. You may then become determined to try a rigid diet to lose weight. As you begin you may find yourself feeling lousy for a while and this could be because you are withdrawing from your daily portion of sugar/fat/salt. If you are not feeling good this will not feel encouraging. After a few days you say "what the hell" and resume your normal eating pattern. Meanwhile you have shamed yourself for not sticking to the diet. Some of these diets will also encourage less carbohydrate, which can decrease the production of serotonin.

At the same time, if you don't address the emotional issues that are contributing to your depression, you will feel the urge to go back to Emotional Eating, even if you do lose the weight. It is easy to feel depressed at our seeming "lack of willpower" when the models or stars in the adverts and other media are so thin, beautiful and so hard to emulate. It's very common to feel inadequate with our rounded, soft bodies if we compare ourselves to these people. But it doesn't mean they aren't Emotional Eaters; when asked, Hannah declared that she definitely wasn't an Emotional Eater, but after a minute she said, ". . . but I don't eat if I am stressed . . ." which says as much about being an Emotional Eater as overeating. It's the very fact that we link food with feelings that creates the strings between us and our relationship with food.

Any of the 7-Day Food Plans will help you with emotional recovery, to fight depression, raise energy levels and help beat stress, but they could also help you to lose weight. When you integrate the Food Plan with the Emotional Eating healing plan you will be on the way to recovery. You will no longer use food to hurt but to heal and nurture your emotional wellbeing.

> It was after I integrated these two ideas that I finally stopped judging myself on how thin I was. I realized that it was feeling physically good that mattered, not how I looked because if I felt physically good, I wasn't always thinking if I looked fat. It took me a long time to get that in my head but it helped me recover from depression.
> MARTINE BUSH, AGED 37

THE EMOTIONAL EATING HEALING PLAN

Here is a ten-point plan to follow in conjunction with one of the 7-Day Food Plans which will offer you a way out from the vicious cycle of Emotional Eating. The steps are meant to be undertaken in order, but it doesn't matter if you mix them up. Take what you want from each step and leave the rest.

It may be that you are a lightweight Emotional Eater; in other words, you know you reach for some chocolate or other rich food when you're stressed and you will succumb to other junk foods when you feel low but, on the whole, Emotional Eating does not rule your physical wellbeing. You may well follow the 80/20 rule: eating good-mood foods 80 percent of the time and submitting to junk for the other 20 percent.

Some of you, however, may feel that Emotional Eating is a way of life and it has taken its toll; you feel tired, stressed, ill and depressed all at the same time and you think this could be something to do with your food. You may follow the 20/80 rule: eating good-mood food for just 20 percent (or less) of the time and junk for the rest.. If this is you, there is a way out.

1. SURRENDER

To begin with, surrender to the fact that you are an Emotional Eater and don't try to fight it.

You may have been on so many "diets" over the years that you don't want one more book telling you what you should be eating because you know what you should be eating. But, damn it, the eating is not the problem! It's why you eat that's become the problem.

Don't start trying to change your food today, because that is an added pressure you can do without. Simply acknowledge that you are an Emotional Eater and you've reached a point where you really want to make some changes to help you feel, and look, better. Don't worry about what you should be eating but simply allow yourself your normal food pattern whilst you come to terms with the whole cycle of Emotional Eating:

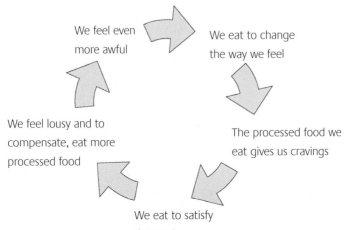

We feel even more awful

We eat to change the way we feel

The processed food we eat gives us cravings

We eat to satisfy the cravings

We feel lousy and to compensate, eat more processed food

Whilst you surrender, become aware of eating the processed foods and how you feel two hours later. Make a mental link between these foods and your feelings, for example:

Food I Eat	How I Feel Two Hours Later
Chips	Headachy
Ice cream	Slightly sinking feeling
Fast-food restaurant burger	Depressed

Don't change your eating patterns whilst you do this; there is no rush. You may have been eating these bad-mood foods for years and it's a positive step to eat the foods whilst watching yourself and objectively noting the different reactions these foods have on your mood. You will become much more sensitive to how these foods affect you rather than making a guess when you are no longer eating them.

Surrender for up to a week, but use each day to immerse yourself in watching your food habits—rather like you were sitting on a stool in the corner and watching yourself; simply raise your awareness. Generally, if we are doing something that is detrimental to us as a way of coping, we really don't like it to be pointed out to us. Denial is a brilliant way to brush aside an ongoing behavior and Emotional Eaters who are in denial, when asked about their Emotional Eating, typically respond:

✳ You think I eat badly, you should see what she eats!
✳ I can diet any time I want, I just don't want to do it now!
✳ I don't eat badly; in fact I'm one of the best eaters I know!
✳ All this talk about food, it's just so boring!

2. IDENTIFY YOUR EMOTIONAL EATING PATTERNS

There may be a pattern around your eating habits; what you eat, when and why. Can you identify them? It's easy to say that you eat simply because you're hungry but as Emotional Eaters there will be added reasons as to why you eat. As you surrender, use this time to note down your patterns, for example:

What I eat	Why I eat it	When I eat it
Chips	Hungry	When I'm without any food
Cakes	Bored	When I get in after work
Chocolate	Makes me feel good	When I'm feeling depressed
Whatever – just lots of it	To punish myself	After I feel bad when I've been with someone I don't like

As you begin to think about your eating patterns, you may identify a blueprint that now seems obvious. For example, you rush in from work, starving, and you dive into the cookie jar to see you through until dinner. Or, you are so hungry you throw a pizza in the microwave to get instant food. Or you eat lots of chocolate if you've had an argument with your partner. At this point, don't judge yourself and don't try to change—the more you simply increase your awareness, the better the long-term results, because you will start to build links between food and emotions and this will help you address your Emotional Eating patterns for the rest of your life.

43 percent of us eat when we feel negative emotions
It is a very common pattern for people to eat when bad emotions arise—in fact 43 percent of us do this and the most common emotion that people eat to stifle is anger. Anger is an extreme emotion that many people seek to avoid feeling. Generally speaking this is because people worry that if they start to express their anger they may "lose control," so they don't get started but instead stifle their feelings. You may have to undertake some form of mood-altering behavior in order to

stifle your anger, because it is a strong emotion and won't go away easily. Typical mood-altering behaviors are smoking, drinking, exercising, working to distraction and eating high-sugar/fat/salt foods.

In undertaking this behavior every time the anger rises to the surface, you can make a good job of keeping it down. However, stifling anger can cause depression and if you couple this with eating "depressive" foods (such as those listed under "Bad-Mood Foods") you can feel really, really bad and sink into a state of misery which is very hard, but not impossible, to climb out of.

If you change your eating "habits" and "food types" you may feel very angry

If your Emotional Eating pattern has led you to stifle your anger with food, but you embark on a smooth, nourishing, whole-food eating plan, like the three plans under the 7-Day Food Plans in Chapter 6, be aware that you may feel the suppressed anger start to rise to the surface. This is very healthy but might be difficult to manage. Concise ways to do this are found in my first book, *Beat Depression and Reclaim Your Life*, but to get started, keep a journal and write down specifics abut how your emotions are changing as your Emotional Eating is changing.

When I started to stop going for the foods that I always craved, particularly chocolate cookies, I started to feel different, emotionally. I began feeling irritable and annoyed at others, so much so that I had to go back to the cookies for a while because it took me by surprise. Then I started again and someone told me that I might feel weird but I felt enraged. I started arguing with people, stamping my foot and generally throwing my weight about like never before. I'm usually a mild person, or so I thought; thank goodness for my tolerant husband. At one point I went into a shop and started complaining in a very heated way about how shoddy the phone was that I had bought and I wasn't budging until they gave me another one. I shouted defiantly at the manager until he told me that I was in the wrong shop! I don't have the anger now and I don't feel depressed either. I've changed my food and my eating habits and I feel in control.

JENNIFER, AGED 29

However, as anger sits on one end of the seesaw, pain is on the other end. You may have to dissolve your anger by reaching the pain to get a good balance in your life. The pain may span many external issues but it always comes down to something you have lost. Begin to identify what sadness is hiding behind your angry feelings and what you have lost.

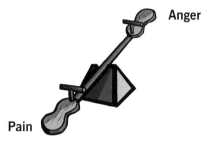

You have to let out anger and pain to get a balance in the seesaw, because a balanced seesaw makes you feel good. Whichever is highest at this moment is the one to concentrate on letting out. In this diagram there is more anger than pain. When the anger starts to be conveyed and heard, the pain will rise up and this may need to be released too. The seesaw will balance out as these emotions are released and a sense of peace will follow.

Draw your own seesaw and define which emotion is more weighted on either side. Next to the seat you can write down what angers you or what you are in pain about. Once these emotions are acknowledged you will find a freedom in yourself and you will have more control over your Emotional Eating patterns.

3. IDENTIFY THE VOICE WHICH CONTROLS YOUR EATING

When we go through the anguish of Emotional Eating habits, there are often two voices in our head and they are battling for top-dog position. These might go something like this:

> *'I know I shouldn't have it but I would love a chocolate bar.'*
> *'Don't have it, you know it will only go on your thighs.'*
> *'Yes, but I feel so good because I did my exercise this morning.'*
> *'Yes, but you will feel bad, emotionally, too.'*
> *'No I won't, because one won't hurt.'*
> *'Remember the old phrase: one is one too many and a thousand never enough.'*
> *'Oh, shut up, I'm going to have it anyway!'*

Does it drive you mad? It drives me mad!

To help quell these voices, one trick is to place "good voice" notes in and around your refrigerator and food cupboards. I know this sounds odd, but it really works. If you have your favorite comfort food in the house, which is too hard to resist in trigger moments, write comforting notes to yourself, appropriate to the food and the trigger, and place them right in front of the food you know you are going to eat under stress. Refer to your hungry heart (see below) and you will know exactly what you need at that moment.

For example, I know that when I have had an argument with my husband, I feel like eating cakes. My husband raises his eyebrows if I eat sugary foods, which is rare, but still, when he does it I go into feeling like a naughty child and damn it—I will eat the cakes! If we don't have any cakes in the house I have been known to drive miles, at 11.30 p.m., to the all-night store and buy some, because my Emotional Eating trigger is so strong.

My problem is that when I get started on high-sugar/fat foods, I can go into trigger overdrive and eat them for days, which I know affects me badly and makes me feel depressed, so I really don't want to even start. Therefore I have learned to temper myself with some warm words written on a couple of notes; one in the cupboard and one in my bag. One note says: "If you eat the cakes you will feel depressed; instead of eating the cakes, express your anger and then go for a run—you will feel GREAT afterwards."

I feel so good if I go with the advice on the note, not just because I feel physically and emotionally good but also because I haven't abused myself.

4. NOURISH THE HUNGRY HEART

Eating to fill the hungry heart is a way of trying to feel more emotionally complete through food. Feeling hollow and empty is a common reason why people eat; it is trying to fill up a hungry heart through food. We are trying to nurture our souls through food and fill the emptiness with doughnuts and potato chips. But food can never fill an empty heart. What we really want is to feel loved and, sometimes, food seems like the easy replacement.

> I am single and lonely but I work hard so I can't get out too much. When I get home, if I feel really lonely I just eat — anything. Before I start I know I'll feel lousy but I do it anyway. It's a vicious circle which I get into and can't get off.
> JOHN, AGED 28

When we Emotionally Eat we tend to eat the foods that cause a depressive mood. This, together with feeling empty and lonely, can send us into a downward spiral. Nevertheless, there are things that you can do to fill up your hungry heart without turning to food.

First, establish whether or not you are eating to feed the hungry heart or whether your Emotional Eating is simply a bad habit. You can do this by asking yourself, when you are hungry, "Am I eating because I feel physically hungry?" or "Am I eating because I am lonely, yearning for company or love?" or "Am I down on myself and I want to feel better?" If you know that you are eating because you're hungry and the cookie you're about to put in your mouth is all you have to hand but you would eat something healthier if it was available, then you are probably simply in a bad habit. If you are longing for something other than food and you think that the cookie will make you "feel better" then you are probably trying to nourish your hungry heart.

Your hungry heart may simply be temporarily depleted of nourishment due to a set of circumstances that have led you to feeling stressed or drained. This could be the result of a divorce or moving house, the loss of a job or illness. If this is the case you may have turned to food as a temporary crutch and now you're reading this book to get yourself back into a sense of rhythm and order.

You may, however, be suffering a deep depression which is the result of profound childhood neglect or deprivation, so your hungry heart has never been properly nourished. You may have always been an Emotional Eater and you are looking for a plan to help you out of the mire and get you living the life that you hear others talk about—a life of self-love and passion where you feel excited about being in this world, relishing each day and feeling liberated and fulfilled. The more unhealed pain you have, the hungrier your heart will be. When your heart is healed, you will no longer feel the pain of its starvation.

To nourish your hungry heart, here is a two-pronged method to approach your Emotional Eating. One is to feed your body with foods that fight depression (see Chapter 5) and the other is to nourish your hungry heart, and here is how.

Find a photo of yourself, or fix an image in your mind, of you when you were younger. Make sure it is a picture of you when you loved yourself and that when you look at it now it makes you feel squishy and soft; you just want to go up to that little girl or boy, pick him up and love him to death.

As you look at the picture, ask yourself what this person needs in order to feel so good that they wouldn't want to do something to themselves to make them feel bad. This may be a big hug, a picnic in the park, some nice words or a day at a theme park! Draw a big heart on a piece of paper and jot down all the things that give you a nice warm feeling in your heart:

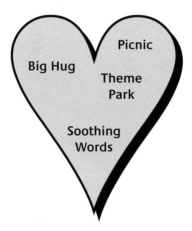

Here are three guiding suggestions:

1. Find ways of immediately fulfilling these desires. If you need a hug, then ask someone for a hug; if no one is available, give yourself a hug or book an appointment with a lovely massage therapist, aromatherapist or someone similar, who can relax you through an hour's blissful touch. If you need a day out at a theme park but you can't do it today, go to the local park and have a big swing but make a date in the diary for when you can get to the theme park. If you want a picnic, just do it. Nice soothing words don't always come from others, so write a letter to yourself and post it, or visit an elderly relative who can ease your worries with kind words!

2. Every time you feel like dashing into the cupboard for a bag of salted nuts, stop and consider that smaller person that you have visualized. If that small person asked you for a hug, would you give her a handful of foods that you knew were going to drain her of energy, make her feel bad and maybe give her a headache? No, you wouldn't; you would probably bend down and give her a big soft hug, ruffle her hair, shower her with kisses and tell her how much you love her because you know she will glow with joy afterwards. This is what you should give yourself if you find yourself dashing to the refrigerator for another lump of cheese.

3. Repeat these simple steps each time that you crave processed foods and you will soon realize a new habit of learning to nourish your hungry heart before you feed your empty stomach. Combining these steps with the food plan to beat depression will help you on your way to feeling so much better.

Whilst I was recovering from depression, I found that the foods I ate and this simple self-talk was enough for me to finally understand how to dispose of the residue of depression that had been hanging around for a couple of years. I look back and wish someone had told me that nourishing the hungry heart before diving into a food substitute could have helped me feel better so much quicker. So even if you have big issues to resolve, you can still undertake these simple steps to gain a positive clarity about your hungry heart.

Of course, some of us have suffered from a deep, devastating depression from which we feel we will never recover. Please take heart, because recovery is possible. If undertaking these steps seems too simple to you, you may need to look at deeper issues, which are covered in my book, *Beat Depression and Reclaim Your Life*. There you will find guidance on how to go about uncovering and healing a lifetime of depression.

5. IDENTIFY THE TRIGGERS

Now you have started to put the brakes on eating depressive foods, you can start to mentally list the triggers that hook you in to an Emotional Eating pattern. Figures show that in spite of all the "healthy" foods available, obesity is growing at an alarming rate. Popular diet plans that help people lose weight often don't help people to keep in shape: up to 95 percent of dieters regain their weight. This is because the Emotional Eating triggers are ignored and when the going gets tough, Emotional Eaters turn to their best friend—comfort food. Once you begin to identify the triggers that set you off, you can start to make lifelong changes that will also address depression and its associated consequences. Here are some examples:

Emotional Eating Trigger	Why
Walking past a burger restaurant	The smell is too hard to resist
Eating with the in-laws	Nervous they will judge me
At home with nothing to do	Haven't had a decent meal
Going to a family function	Always winds me up so I deal with it by eating junk

The Emotional Eating triggers are usually obvious when you begin to note them down, and once they're identified it becomes very simple to begin a pattern of change. For example, if you can't resist food from a particular restaurant, walk down another road; the smell is deliberately there to entice you in. If you are eating with the in-laws, discuss your nervousness with your spouse or partner before you go—this will help you feel supported. If you're at home and eating through boredom, leaf through some delicious recipes and start cooking—remember, good home-cooked food is going to help you to beat depression better than snacking.

Finally, if being with your family still causes you anxiety as an adult, take a look at some historic issues which may be still bothering you. It may not just be the issues between you and your family, but some of the messages you picked up in your family while you were growing up.

All the time I was growing up I heard my mother say she couldn't eat "stodge" as she called it. When I ate a pudding I felt so bad because she would sit and not eat it. Instead she would smoke at the table. I got the feeling that I shouldn't be eating stodge either, but I loved it. As I got older I became secretive about eating stodge until I started to steal cookies and chocolate and then hide them. It wasn't the eating it that affected me as much as my behavior around the stodge stuff. As an adult I have had to calm myself down around puddings, as I used to get so anxious eating sweet stuff around my family and either tended to ignore the puddings or stuff my face, and I couldn't find a way to be calm around my family with a meal happening too. But I feel much more level now and, as a result, I simply don't crave the sweet stuff.

SHARON, AGED 39

6. GREAT CRAVING SUBSTITUTES

While hunger can be satisfied by any half-decent meal, food cravings are specific and immediate. Almost all of us get cravings. Yet guilt follows us when we have filled our stomach with whatever food had that hold on us. Of course, if your craving is a green apple it may not affect your overall health. But if you would kill for a burger and fries every day, you may harm yourself physically and emotionally.

There are no obvious clues as to why we get cravings and little research to explain their power over us. If it were simply a nutritional deficiency then we could take a pill to alleviate that deficiency, like a pill containing magnesium instead of a bar of chocolate (which contains magnesium). But it's not that simple. It's more an Emotional Eating pattern—a reaction to circumstance, rather than a depletion of a nutrient.

It's also not any good anyone telling you not to crave your favorite "got to have it" food because, like an addict, you will pay no attention. However, there are certain foods which may help with certain cravings and will reduce the depressing effect that craving foods might have.

Craving For	Gotta Have	Great Substitute
Chocolate	Dairy milk chocolate bar	70% chocolate – 4 squares hits the spot!
Ice cream	Thick and rich, creamy and gooey ice cream	Frozen yogurt – one scoop satisfies
Salt snack	Bag of salted peanuts	Natural peanut butter spread on whole-grain toast – fills you up too
Cake	Anything with icing	Tell yourself you'll have it after an apple; the apple will massively reduce your sugar craving
Anything, because I'm starving, in town and gotta to eat before I get home	Cheese and ham sandwich with mustard and pickle	Get the packaged sushi – fish or vegetarian – from a supermarket; filling and more wholesome than a white-bread and cheese sandwich
Chips	Salt and vinegar	Make some popcorn – 2 tbsp heated olive oil, 1 layer popcorn and heat until all the corn is popped.
Cookie	Chocolate chip	Handful of raw nuts (toasted if you prefer)
Sugar	Candy	Banana – helps cut the craving dead
Alcohol	Glass of wine	Go for a walk, run, or even "stepping" on the stairs first, promising yourself that drink when you get back – your craving will be reduced

7. THREE MEALS A DAY

"Three Meals a Day" can bring calm into your Emotional Eating. When we are depressed our lives can become chaotic and unruly. This does nothing but add to our distress. By introducing "Three Meals a Day" we can implement a simple but effective way of self-managing our unmanageable life.

"Three Meals a Day" is simply that—eating three meals in a given day: breakfast, lunch and dinner. To the uninitiated, this may seem like a task too simple and too obvious, but to those of us who have suffered depression, eating regular meals can come way down on the list of priorities. Not only does eating three meals a day have wonderful repercussions on your physical health (see Chapter 2) but it also gives a sense of flow and order to your life, which can help bring about emotional stability. Many depressed people will simply grab food as they go or pay little attention to their nutritional needs and quickly find themselves feeling lethargic, depressed and stressed without realizing how their Emotional Eating is causing this.

So what does "Three Meals a Day" mean? It means that we will respect ourselves enough to plan, prepare and nourish our emotional wellbeing by eating a regular pattern of good-mood foods that will help us feel more steady and constant. Feeling this way is a good starting point for beating depression by offering us the end of the tangled ball of string in which our emotions are all jumbled. Finding one focal point from which we can expand outwards can give us optimism and release from the hopelessness that comes with depression.

As you embark on this new way of eating, you may find it hard to stick at to begin with. Don't be alarmed. You may have to do several things to bring about good changes. Here are some guidelines:

✷ Firstly you may get craving for the foods to which you turn to nourish your heart when you are feeling depressed. Don't be rigid but simply eat half the amount of processed foods that you ate yesterday. You will then have fewer cravings.

✻ Unfamiliar emotions may surface. If you are prepared for them you will not be flummoxed. These emotions are what you have suppressed through Emotional Eating and they have to come up and out for you to heal.

✻ One emotion that may surface is guilt; guilt for eating at all, and this may be prevalent around breakfast time because breakfast can seem so unnecessary to an Emotional Eater who eats on the run. However, it is the most important meal because it can help your blood-sugar levels smooth out so the emotional swings may be curtailed. See "Breakfast For All" in Chapter 6 for some good ideas.

✻ Get some support if you need it. Overeaters Anonymous (www.oa.org) is a 12-Step support group that is full of people who are stabilizing their Emotional Eating.

As you settle into this routine you will begin to notice positive changes in your relationship with food. Here are a few examples:

✻ You will feel more nourished and balanced
✻ You will feel happier
✻ You will enjoy your food more
✻ You will see food less as a threat
✻ You will feel more cared for
✻ You will feel more in control
✻ You will probably lose weight if you are overweight

8. THE FIVE RULE

As we have already seen, the Five Rule is eating a minimum of five portions of fruit and vegetables every day.

Fruit and vegetables are full of depression-busting, immune-system boosting, digestion-aiding, cleansing and mood-enhancing nutrients that we just don't want to be without. By ensuring that we receive these foods we are one step further in nourishing our physical and emotion wellbeing. By making the effort to ensure these powerful foods are included in our diet, we are implementing positive changes toward fighting depression.

When I asked various people the question: "How many portions of fruit and vegetables do you have a day?" their responses included: sometimes; never; I try but it's too much effort; do fries count? We are not in the habit of ensuring we are following the Five Rule and it can seem hard work to get in the habit. But if you want to feel less depressed then use one of the 7-Day Food Plans—these will help you get your Five a Day. All you have to do is follow the plan and you don't even need to think about it.

The other side of the coin is that you will naturally eat less "depressing" foods. By adding the Five Rule you will automatically ditch some of the processed foods. Chapter 6 looks at snacks that follow the Five Rule and if you follow some of these ideas, not only will you get the strength of the natural whole foods, you will get fewer cravings for the highly processed foods.

9. HEALING FOODS

Learn to love your food through healing foods. Healing food is food that is closer to its original structure than processed food. Think of healing foods as "genesis" foods; whole grains, fresh vegetables, brown rice, fresh fruit, beans, fish, etc. As you eat more healing foods you will be loving the food you eat, because they are just that, they love your body, they heal your body and in turn you will love yourself.

The more healing foods you eat, the more you love your food and yourself. It can't be any other way; that is the power of food. The positive effect that healing foods have on your body will help you to fight depression, stress and fatigue; it will also help you to contain your Emotional Eating.

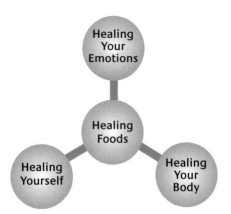

Healing foods have their opposite, and they are "hurting foods." These are far from their origins—the earth—and can hurt our mind, body and spirit. They are foods which deplete us of energy because the body is using much of its energy to try and minimize the harm that hurting foods do to us. In eating them we have less regard for the healing foods and more cravings and desire for the processed foods, which are high in fat/sugar/salt and are whiter in color. The more processed the food, the less likely it is to support you emotionally. This may seem like a wild generalization but if you find yourself debating your meal, think genesis or earth foods for better emotional wellbeing and you will come closer to healing foods.

When I first looked at the 7-Day Food Plan for Depression I thought, "Oh, no!"—brown, raw-ish type of foods! Then I twigged. I usually eat processed foods and this was maybe why I was feeling so depressed. After finishing the week's food plan, I felt so much better but what made me realize just how much better I felt was when I ate a burger in a bap at a fair. The fat dribbled down my arm to my elbow and I was disgusted but starving. I ate it and an hour later I burst into tears because it made me feel so bad! I do anything to make sure I stick to brown foods now and, strangely enough, my confidence has zoomed.

NATALIE, AGED 32

Healing foods vs hurting foods

HEALING FOODS Genesis foods	HURTING FOODS Processed foods
Whole-grain bread	White bread
Whole-grain pasta	White pasta
Brown rice / lentils	White rice
Dark honey	Sugar
Tomato sauce	Cheese sauce
Berries	Cookies
Baked potatoes	French fries
Olive oil	Butter / margarine
Herbs	Salt
Dark greens	Baked beans
Red apples	Candy
Beetroot	Potato Chips
Lean meat	Sausages
Raspberry sauce	Cream
Blackcurrant sorbet	Vanilla ice cream

10. GRIEVE YOUR LOSSES

The final step is to allow yourself to grieve the losses that your Emotional Eating has been suppressing. Allow the hungry heart pain to rise to the surface and release it. As we discussed under the Five Rule, you may experience emotions that rise up which have been suppressed through Emotional Eating. But, you may also grieve the loss of food as your support.

Consider what part Emotional Eating has played in your life. Has food been your best friend? Has it been your lover? It may have become your enemy with which you have fought a long and bloody war! By identifying what Emotional Eating has represented, you will be able to find ways of replacing food with new tools. You can say goodbye to the control food has had over you as you finally gain control over what you eat. You may have used food as a way of coping through a relationship break-up, and now you feel it's time to replace the food with some alternative method of support.

Saying goodbye to food as your crutch can be like saying goodbye to an abusive love partner. You love them but hate them. You know you're better off without them but you will still miss them. They may have harmed you but they were the only ones there for you. You can learn from how it was and how you never want to go there again. Just as you still need people, so you still need to eat, but your whole approach to eating can change for the better and can change your life in a powerful and positive way.

Saying goodbye

You can write a letter to your old food tendencies and thank the food for how it has supported you for so long. You can outline how you are going to replace Emotional Eating to nourish your hungry heart and what you are going to gain as a result. In this letter you can outline your goals and desires with a timescale. Keep this letter close to your heart and if ever you need to understand why you have made these changes, you have the substantiation to look back on and take strength from.

> Since I have taken control of my life through better eating, I have a new life. I used to feel wretched most days but now I have purpose. I have beaten depression for life.
> SUE SWAIN, AGED 61

4
BAD-FOOD FALLOUT

Does bad food cause depression? There is no doubt about it! Your body is like a high-performance car and you can't afford to give it anything less than the best maintenance in order to keep it running smoothly and without a hiccup. With a high-performance car you have to ensure that it is regularly tuned, the tires are checked, oil filter replaced, brake pads tested and emissions checked in order for it to drive you safely and securely. However, if you omit these basics and fill it with the incorrect fuel or neglect the tires, the car will start to jangle, stall and not perform to its potential.

Your body is no different. We all know how awful a hangover feels or how stuffed and lethargic we feel when we've had a "blowout" meal. It is more difficult to notice the different performance in your body when you deplete your diet of goodness over a longer period of time. But this is what happens when you don't regularly maintain your body with the nutrients it needs to function at an optimum level. In fact, there are very direct consequences of eating the wrong foods, which can produce depressing reactions in our bodies.

TOP 5 'BAD-MOOD FOODS'

The amount of information we receive about foods and their effect on our bodies leaves us unclear and confused, because there is so much opinion and a lot less hard facts. However, there are five specific foods that unquestionably cause a "bad-mood food" impact on the body and they are listed below.

1. SALT – THE SLUG KILLER

Too much salt inhibits good kidney function and unhappy kidneys can lead to depression and fatigue. Have you ever tried the age-old "natural" remedy for ridding your garden of slugs?

It's the treatment which involves placing salt in the area where slugs appear last thing at night. Have you seen the results the next morning? The slugs are dead, they have sores all over them and their bodies have gone into a strange shape like a corkscrew (similar to those twisted chips you can buy) as the hydration has defeated them.

This is what happens to our kidneys when we eat too much salt. We need our kidneys to feel energetic, and if our kidneys can't do their job we end up feeling enervated, we suffer lower-back pain, experience feeble knees and we have to keep going to the toilet because our bladder is weak. Usually the salt is deposited in the joints, particularly the knees, which may result later in arthritis and rheumatism. It makes no difference where the salt has come from, for instance table salt, sea salt or processed foods; the results are the same. If our kidneys are not functioning adequately, we do not feel good and not feeling good on a long-term basis can lead to a depressed mood.

On average we eat around 9–12g of salt a day. Government guidelines tell us not to have more than **6g of salt** a day (a flat teaspoon). Three-quarters of the salt we eat comes from processed food, such as breakfast cereals, soups, sauces, ready meals, cookies etc., and almost everyone eats some processed foods. Even people who make all their own meals from scratch will usually buy foods such as bread and cookies, which can be high in salt. Taking this into account, we should only add a further **1.5g extra** of salt per day to our cooking, which is about the same weight as a paperclip or the amount found in one slice of bread.

According to the British Nutrition Foundation (BNF), if we were to reduce salt intake to 6g a day, about 20 percent fewer people would get strokes and 15 percent fewer would get heart attacks. In fact, the BNF has calculated that if we were to go on a diet consisting purely of natural meats, fruits and vegetables, with no salt added, our sodium intake would drop by 80 to 85 percent. Of course, we add salt to food, but this accounts only for a surprising 15 to 20 percent of the salt we consume in total. This huge intake of salt is contributing to our stress, lethargy and depression.

So, how do we cut down on salt? The key to success is to do this slowly. Unlike losing weight, giving up smoking or getting fit, reducing salt intake gradually is completely painless.

❋ **Firstly**, start by omitting salt from the cooking process. We are so used to putting salt into a pan of water to cook our vegetables to give that extra "vroom" or throwing in a large pinch of salt to a sauce. It is a habit we have learned, but it is not necessary to the cooking process. By eliminating this added salt we can gently begin to reduce our intake. The difference in taste will not be that noticeable and after a couple of weeks your palate will have adapted to eating less salt.

❋ **Secondly**, forget to purchase salt for the table when you next run out. Shaking salt over a meal can provide as much as 5g of salt in one shot. This can be eliminated, but if you have already eradicated salt in cooking, shaking salt onto food will begin to taste unpleasant. If you receive howls of complaint from a partner or family, plead stupidity/ignorance and explain you forgot the salt again! Keep this up and after three weeks have gone by, they will have probably stopped asking you and you will have all got used to not grinding the salt mill over your meals. Once you have accomplished the first two steps, you're almost there!

❋ **Thirdly**, look at processed foods. Seventy-five percent of the foods we buy are processed, and 75 percent of our salt intake comes from processed foods, so it makes sense to keep an eye on exactly what salt content is in these foods. Sodium is another word for salt and is often used instead of salt on food labels. High levels of salt can turn up in unexpected places other than the obvious cakes, pastries and cookies—it's also found in foods such as bread and breakfast cereals. Basically, if a food is packaged then it has had salt added to it. Food labels will tell you how much salt a food contains, but they can be difficult to understand. If you are confused, look for the salt content per 100g of the food. For comparison think of seawater: if your food says more than 1.25g sodium per 100g food, then the food has more salt than seawater! Would you drink seawater?

As your palate changes and you become used to taking in less salt, you will naturally lean toward less salty foods. As the salt cravings diminish, the body will actually find salty foods to be quite offensive.

Meanwhile, there are some ways to spice up the mildness in your food when you begin to reduce salt in your cooking. Start by marinating food before cooking it. Here are some examples:

* an olive oil, garlic and fresh basil mash is a delicious and rich blend for a chicken marinade
* coconut milk and crushed cilantro is a mouth-watering combination for fish
* some honey, chopped thyme and a dash of vinegar is a delicious way to cook lamb

Some other ideas to liven up food:
* add chopped chives to mashed potatoes
* include chopped celery in with dishes that require onions
* throw in chopped parsley to rice dishes
* make a rich tomato sauce by simmering a can of chopped tomatoes and adding some tomato purée to taste, a crushed garlic clove and a dash of balsamic vinegar
* drizzle lemon juice and/or olive oil over vegetables
* discover the power of ginger in Thai or Indian meals
* add toasted pine nuts, pumpkin or sesame seeds to salad dishes
* melt goats' cheese onto roast vegetables

❋ add a spoon of natural peanut butter to a stir-fry
❋ discover a home-made curry powder or paste
❋ melt home-made garlic butter onto vegetables

2. BAD-MOOD FATS

As a nation, we love fries. And we love fried chicken, deep-fried potato skins. And we adore doughnuts, cookies, cakes and pastries, especially when the smell wafts out from the bakery section. What makes them taste so good? They all contain saturated and trans fats and this is what gives them that delicious, rich, mouth-watering, mood-altering, fatty taste. It's the good, the bad and the ugly all rolled into one: they taste delicious but we know they are bad for our health. Did you also know that they can really affect the way you feel and deplete you of energy, brightness and a bountiful mood?

For years we have heard how bad saturated fats are for us. There is a whole host of research backing up how saturated fats raise our levels of cholesterol and consequently block our arteries, which may give rise to heart disease. More recently there has been a lot of attention on trans-fatty acids and although more research is to be done, it is clear that this type of fat also has a role to play in raising cholesterol and creating as many arterial problems as saturated fats. But what the research hasn't focused on is how eating these types of fats can depress the mood, and create sluggishness and tiredness.

Bad-mood fats such as saturated and trans fats are a toxin to the body and when the body is assaulted with toxins it will create mucus to try and eliminate them. If we catch a cold the body will produce a lot of mucus, which results in plenty of coughing and blowing the nose. The toxins are expelled with the mucus. In the same vein, when we eat lots of saturated fats our body will accept these fats as a toxin and will produce mucus as a defense mechanism.

An overload of mucus can give you a woolly feeling like a "head cold," leaving you feeling blocked up or congested. When you are depressed there is nothing worse than this feeling, and it can easily leave you feeling even more dispirited, lethargic and without any energy.

Another reason why saturated fats can make you depressed is because of the excessive levels of triglyceride found in blood fat high in cholesterol. Research undertaken in 1994 by Charles Glueck, MD, Medical Director of the Cholesterol Center of Jewish Hospital in Cincinnati, USA, found that high cholesterol levels are not only bad for the heart, they're dreadful for the brain. High blood levels of cholesterol, and especially triglycerides, are strongly correlated with the frequency of affective disorders including depression, manic depression, and schizoaffective disorder as well as with hostility and aggression. Most fats in food are composed of triglycerides, which are broken down to various fatty acids. "We have shown that in patients with high triglycerides who were in a depressive state, the more you lower the triglycerides, the more you alleviate the depression."

In order to feel better it's a good time to look at the amount of saturated and trans fats in your diet and change what you are eating to make a powerful change in your mood. But where do you start? There is so much information about fats that it is hard to sift the nuggets from it. Here is a summary:

Bad fats

Trans Fats: Trans fats were invented by scientists to "hydrogenate" liquid oils so that they could perform better in the food production process and provide a better shelf life. The "hydrogenation" is a technique to make liquid fats into solid fats, with hydrogen, and so easier to cook with. As a result of hydrogenation, trans-fatty acids are formed. Trans-fatty acids are found in many commercially packaged goods and in most processed foods or junk foods. Indeed, "low fat" or "healthy option" foods contain significant amounts of trans fats and you cannot avoid them if you eat cookies, cakes, chocolate bars, sweet bars, cookies, commercially fried food or use margarines and margarine spreads.

Saturated Fats: Saturated fats raise total blood cholesterol as well as LDL cholesterol (the bad cholesterol). Saturated fats are mainly found in animal products such as meat, dairy, eggs and seafood. Some plant foods are also high in saturated fats such as coconut, palm oil and palm kernel oil.

Good fats
Goods fats are healthy. They don't raise cholesterol in the same way as saturated fats. In fact, studies are now suggesting that these oils, but particularly olive oil, can actually decrease the amount of cholesterol in the body. The US Food and Drug Administration (FDA), in November 2004, stated that "using two tablespoons of olive oil per day in place of other fats may be enough to produce this LDL-lowering effect so our arteries have a better chance of staying clear." An FDA statement is one to be taken seriously, and so by pouring olive oil over food on a regular basis may give us a chance to undo some of the bad-mood fat effects.

Here is a list of all the good-mood fats:
* oily fish
* avocados
* nuts and seeds
* sunflower, rapeseed and olive oil and spreads
* vegetable oils

Did you know that 25 years ago olive oil was only available from the pharmacist?

How to increase the good fats and decrease the bad fats to fight depression

Labels: The very first thing you can do is check the labels as you shop. However, labels can be nightmare, because although they are supposed to be there to help guide us through the maze of nutritional know-how, we are discovering that they can blind us with it as well. For instance, low fat doesn't mean "low fat." As a rough guide, the World Health Organization suggests we should have no more than 30 percent of our diet as fat. But for optimum mental health, it would be prudent to aim for no more than 10 percent of your diet being saturated fat. Although saturated fats have to be listed, to date trans fats don't, which is a huge criticism considering these fats may be the worse thing in the foodstuff for your good mental health! So look out for—and avoid—hydrogenated vegetable fats! Go for monounsaturated and polyunsaturated fats, which are beneficial as they help lower blood cholesterol levels.

Some food substitutes
* oily fish instead of sausages or a meat pie
* For cooking, use olive oil instead of butter, margarine or lard in cooking
* snack on some unsalted nuts or seeds instead of a biscuit or cake
* make your mashed potato with olive oil and garlic instead of butter and milk for a change

Ace Butter: What is the answer when it comes to spreads? For years we've heard that butter is full of saturated fats and spreads are filled with trans fats. If you simply love a little butter on your vegetables and you cannot do without it, here is a good middle-ground option—Ace Butter. This is a quick recipe to make up which will take you five minutes and resolve your conscience:

Ace Butter ingredients
½ cup olive oil
¾ cup butter

Method: Gently melt the butter in a heavy saucepan but don't allow it to separate. Once melted, add the olive oil. Put into a dish to set and place in the refrigerator.

Do not enter

The very worst thing you can eat to encourage a depressive mood is trans fat. This is apparent when fats are heated to a high temperature, over and over again. You can actually smell bad trans fats before you go into a restaurant or kitchen. It's a slightly rancid smell and you will know exactly what it is once you've smelled it.

3. THE DAIRY TRAIN

How do dairy foods impact on our mood? We have been brought up to assume that milk and its by-products are good for us. A warm glass of milk before bed is nurturing, a chunk of cheese with some bread is a regular snack, and a cream cake is a gorgeous treat. But what is the downside?

High fat, high fatigue

Firstly, dairy products are high in saturated fats, which can increase blood cholesterol and cause poor circulation to the brain, inhibiting the synthesis of neurotransmitters. As these neurotransmitters, such as serotonin, play such a vital role in the way we feel, any malfunction in their performance will negatively impact on our mood.

High cholesterol is also associated with an increased risk of heart disease because it causes damage to, and a narrowing of, the arteries. When the arteries are narrowed, they may become incapable of supplying enough blood and oxygen to the heart muscle during exertion and oxygen deprivation causes muscle pain, fatigue and "brain fog." We know we shouldn't pour hot fats down the sink because, when they hit the cooler fluids, they will block up the pipes and cause an obstruction. Fats can clog our bodies up in a similar way.

The dairy high

Secondly, the foods we turn to when we feel depressed can often contain high levels of dairy foods—cheese, milkshakes, creamy soups and sauces, ice creams etc. These foods are hard to knock on the head when we feel dejected or down in the dumps, and sometimes they are the only source of comfort. But they also contain many of the other five "bad-mood foods" (sugar, salt, trans fats and refined carbohydrates) so not only are you eating foods that are renowned for clogging your blood channels, you are also adding the drawbacks of other ingredients and very likely bypassing the good-mood boosters like fresh fruit, pulses or vegetables.

So by decreasing the amount of dairy products you eat you are quite likely to decrease the amount of bad-mood foods as well.

The osteoporosis/depression issue

Something else is bubbling in the pot. A study at the Harvard Medical School which followed more than 75,000 women for 12 years showed that increased milk consumption—and hence increased intake of calcium—far from protecting against fracture risk was in fact associated with a higher fracture risk. Other studies have backed up this data and have shown that you can actually decrease your risk of osteoporosis by reducing your dairy intake.

How can this be? Well, dairy products are not a natural food for humans. We are the only species that continues to consume milk after we have been weaned and we drink the milk intended for a dissimilar species. The problem is that protein in dairy products creates strong acids in the bloodstream that the body needs to work hard at to neutralize. It will take calcium from the bones to help neutralize the acidity levels. And, because skimmed and semi-skimmed milk has less fat, it contains more protein and the liver needs to work even harder and requires more calcium from the bones. The harder the liver has to work, the more likely you are to gain bad-food fallout.

Once osteoporosis is diagnosed, you may be offered HRT to increase bone density, and the side effects of HRT can include depression, fatigue, headaches, breast tenderness, premenstrual syndrome, skin irritation and weight gain. Added to that, there is a link between bone thinning and depression and it is thought that major depression is associated with hormonal abnormalities that can lead to changes in tissue such as bone. Research carried out by the National Institute of Mental Health in Maryland suggests that higher cortisol levels, often found in depressed patients, may contribute to bone loss and changes in body composition. It therefore makes sense to combat any chance of this link by weaning yourself off the dairy and sourcing calcium intake through other means.

Foods with a high calcium content include kale, greens, dried figs, broccoli or pilchards in tomato sauce.

The good news

The good news is that once you start to decrease your intake of dairy fats, you should start to feel less fatigue and depression and, because of the wonderful benefits of replacement foods, you could start to feel lighter and cleaner, and this will help to brighten your mood.

Here are some wonderful foods to help wean you off the dairy:

High Dairy Foods	Replace with
Hard cheese	Pecorino Romano cheese — similar to Parmesan but made from sheep's milk and can be used to flavor pastas or on a cheese board with some grapes.
Soft cheese	Goats' cheese — a clean, subtle cheese, delicious on its own or melted over some roasted root vegetables. Cottage cheese is the best dairy cheese replacement; just check its salt levels.
Cream	Almond cream is divine as a cream substitute for desserts. Just don't go there!
Ice cream	Fruit sorbets are the perfect replacement and taste even better than ice cream.
Milk	If you want an alternative there are some brilliant milks made from rice, almonds and soya.
Yogurt	The new types of soya yoghurts are gorgeous, but make them plain and add your own fruit.
Butter	If you love a little butter with your vegetables, try the Ace Butter recipe (see page 86). Oil is a great substitute for cooking — use olive for savories and sunflower for sweet recipes.

All of the 7-Day Food Plans will offer a good opening for eating with a limited dairy intake and they will help you to gain more energy and fight depression and fatigue.

4. OUR DAILY BREAD

"And Give Us This Day Our Daily Bread . . ."? But make it whole grain!

White bread is a bona fide promoter of depression. It is made from stripped, white flour, which is a refined carbohydrate with a sky-high GI factor. White flour is so refined that it has been milled and robbed of its original, natural elements such as fiber, healthy oils, vitamins and minerals. This refined carbohydrate is so depleted of any nutrients that bakeries are required by law to add calcium and B-vitamins.

The GI factor

This highly deprived product plays havoc on our digestive system and on our mood. The refined carbohydrates release their sugar quickly into the blood, causing a dramatic rise in insulin, which has the same affect as a "sugar rush" and will leave you feeling tired and lethargic.

Measuring the GI factor of your bread will help you to eat better mood-building foods. The GI (glycemic index) factor is a way of measuring how fast a food converts to sugar in the body. If a food converts quickly, it is a high-GI food, for example white bread; if it converts slowly, it has a low GI rating, like berries. This is important if you suffer from depression, because when your body produces sugar too rapidly it causes a sudden flood of unnatural glucose by releasing large amounts of insulin into the bloodstream. You will feel the initial "rush" of energy followed by a "crash" later on. This is a cause of depression and is best avoided to enable a beneficial and stable mood.

Have you ever had a sandwich for lunch, made with white bread, and then felt as though you needed an afternoon nap because you were so tired? That is probably a lot to do with the white bread that you ate. An hour later, you just have to have a cookie or piece of cake when your energy levels are at their lowest? That's the "carb connection."

Where's all the good fiber gone?

White bread has had most of its fiber removed. The gorgeous husk and wheat germ of the grain is no longer present and this makes a slice of white bread a very difficult food to navigate through the stomach. Put a slice of white bread in a large glass of water and watch it expand to the edge of the glass and turn into a gooey, glutinous mess. This is what the body has to cope with. Lack of fiber in white bread can cause constipation, which is a horrible condition leaving the sufferer feeling irritable, tired, sluggish and generally miserable. In addition, white flour is so stripped of the natural selenium and oils that come from the ground that we don't receive the essential food mood boosters that come from whole foods. It is also deficient in chromium (essential for blood-sugar control), zinc, iron and B-vitamins, which are immune boosters and depression busters.

Malnourishment and irritability

Deficiency in zinc, iron and B-vitamins were implicated in a 14-year study concluded in 2004, examining the links between childhood diet and antisocial behavior as teenagers. Compared to those with a healthy diet, malnourished children showed a 51 percent rise in aggression at 17. According to Professor Adrian Raine of the University of Southern California, "Poor nutrition characterized by zinc, iron, vitamin B and protein deficiencies leads to low IQ, which leads to later antisocial behavior. These are all nutrients linked to brain development." Similar conclusions were drawn from a 2002 study of young offenders at Aylesbury prison in the UK whose diet was supplemented with vitamins and essential fatty acids. Antisocial behavior fell by 35 percent. So if you feel dense and irritable, take a look at your white bread.

It's not just bread

Of course, these problems are not confined to bread—white pasta, rice and all other products that are stripped of their natural fiber can leave us feeling depressed and tired. Cakes, cookies, pastries, sausage rolls, pasties, cookies, doughnuts, etc., all present the same difficulties for our bodies. Some of these products have the added sugar, trans fats and salt that really can hit our mood badly. If we suffer from depression, we really want to avoid foods that will make it worse.

So, what's the answer?

Whole grains!

Yes, they can seem hard to swallow to begin with, but here's a promise: when you gradually change over to whole-grain foods, you will start to feel better. Once you begin to feel better you will appreciate how whole grains have had a big part to play and this could well motivate you to eat more whole grains and gradually ditch the white flour

* BREAD: the terms you want to look for are "whole wheat" or "whole grain" breads. This means that the whole grain has been used. Look for lower-GI breads—the best variety are the coarse grain varieties: stone-ground, wholewheat, wholemeal pitta and rye.
* PASTA: whole-grain or wholewheat pasta; the new whole-grain pastas coming onto the market are great. There was a time when whole-grain spaghetti tasted like a soggy, cardboard box, but no longer; they are also no more expensive.
* RICE: brown rice is the way to go. Again, like pasta, this rice used to be like eating budgerigar droppings, but they are now more delicious and nutty than white rice.

It's that simple: switch from white to brown products and you could immediately elevate your energy levels and boost your mood.

5. AS SWEET AS SUGAR?

One of the main "bad-mood foods" that impacts on depression is sugar. The sugar you buy in the supermarket is an unnatural substance processed from natural sugar beet and refined down to a pure sucrose which has no nutritional value whatsoever. This pure sucrose is said to be akin to a toxin to the human body, because the body is just not able to handle the amounts of sugar we now consume. It is estimated that in the West every man, woman and child ingests a teaspoon of sugar every half an hour—24 hours a day.

What happens when you eat sugar? Since all carbohydrates need specific nutrients (vitamins B1, B2, B3, B5, B6 and magnesium) to be properly digested in the body and since refined sugars are devoid of such nutrients, these must be obtained from bodily reserves, thus depleting these reserves and causing marginal nutritional deficiency, which is a contributor to generally feeling lousy.

The sugar rush

When we eat sugar and we feel that "sugar rush," the body is trying to compensate for the large amount of unnatural glucose it has received by releasing sizeable amounts of insulin into the bloodstream. This has the effect of making you feel "high" for a short while and is often mistaken for a spurt of "energy." However, within an hour or two you will feel the downside because your blood-sugar level crashes and you feel listless, tired and depressed. You may then look for another "quick fix" to help you over the down patch by eating another cake or bar of chocolate, and so the cycle continues. Many people who are diagnosed with depression also discuss their "sugar addiction."

Our bodies can only cope with the onslaught of sugar overdosing for so long and this has had a big impact on the huge rise of type-2 diabetes, which is said to be growing at 15 percent a year.

The National Institute of Diabetes and Digestive and Kidney Diseases (NIDDK) estimates that 20.8 million people—7 percent of the US population—had diabetes in 2005. People with diabetes have a higher-than-average rate of depression; is this because they eat a lot of sugar or because diabetes causes depression? No one knows, but it is worth cutting back on, if not cutting out, sugar.

The good news is that, just like with salt, eating sugar is simply a habit that can be changed, and by changing this one habit, you will start to boost your mood. By reducing your sugar intake, you will reduce your cravings for that sugar "high" and, conversely, as you reduce your cravings you will gain more energy that doesn't require a sugar fix to get you started. The two areas to concentrate on are the hidden sugar in your food and the sugar you put onto your food.

Hidden sugars

In the last two decades, sugar consumption has increased by 31 percent, to 1.25lb (over half a kilo) per person per week. Though fewer and fewer of us take sugar in our coffee, and sprinkle less over our cereals and desserts, we are actually consuming more.

When you begin to read labels on foodstuffs, you may find they can be difficult to understand, but you will soon begin to interpret them. Ingredients that end in "ose," such as dextrose, fructose or sucrose, are different kinds of sugars, and honey, molasses, sorbitol, mannitol and corn syrup are also sugars and add to the sugar content of a product. If one of the first three ingredients listed on the label is a sugar, then you may take it as read that the sugar content of that product is very high. If a product says it is unsweetened it usually means that no sugar or sweetener has been added to the food, but it doesn't mean that it contains no sugar. Also, be wary of "healthy" products as they are prone to be misleading. For instance, the fruit variety "bio" yoghurts that you find on the shelves appear as "healthy" but can contain up to 15 percent sugar.

Added sugar

If you want to satisfy your sweet tooth but don't want the depressive fallout effect from sugar, then try these suggestions:

✻ Start by halving the amount of sugar you currently use: use half the amount in your tea and coffee, on your cereal, in your cooking and when sprinkling over fruits and other foods
✻ Eating something crunchy is said to have a good effect on your sugar craving
✻ Grab a handful of raw nuts if you feel peckish
✻ Replace sugary puddings with plain yoghurt and fresh fruit
✻ If you need to make a dessert, steer toward fruit puddings and away from sponges, chocolate and creamy desserts, which all have a high sugar count
✻ Add fruit toppings for waffles or pancakes instead of syrups or treacle (a dollop of stewed berries on a waffle is sumptuous)
✻ Add spices to fruit and other desserts to lessen your need for sugar; it's a different taste but just as delicious (cinnamon is lovely with apples and ginger is gorgeous with bananas).
✻ If you have a sugar craving, eat sweet fruit such as mangos, pineapple or ripe pears
✻ Make a pure fruit sorbet and sweeten it with canned fruit in its own juice.

All these tips will help to reduce your sugar cravings and, over time, you will feel less like eating sugar. Juliet Hart, an avid healthy eater who has avoided eating sugar for several years, says, "Not only has this beaten my depression but I have such sensitive taste buds now that I can taste sugar in an instant. It's become a bit of a game; if my husband and I eat out, I can tell immediately whether or not a savory dish served in a restaurant has sugar in it, because I will feel the 'sugar high' immediately and then slightly dazed after about twenty minutes." For Juliet it was necessary to simply stop eating sugar altogether because even a small amount would heighten her craving for more so much that she wouldn't be able to resist.

Since stopping eating sugar, she has come off antidepressants and no longer suffers prolonged periods of depression.

TEN COMMON BAD-MOOD FOOD FALLOUTS

Below are some of the common "fallout" symptoms that can arise as a result of eating the wrong foods. All of these problems are exasperated by a poor diet low on fresh foods and high in processed foods, but there are some specific links between these problem areas and certain foods, and these are highlighted.

By omitting some of the above top five "Bad-Mood Foods" and replacing them with alternatives to support your body, you will help it to build itself back to good emotional health and will rapidly feel the rewards of your efforts. Let's now look at some other ways we can target specific areas which might exasperate, contribute to, or even cause depression, and discuss foods to help turn these symptoms around so that we feel good.

1. CHRONIC FATIGUE

Chronic fatigue is a condition which manifests itself as a persistent state of exhaustion. The early signs are a strong and noticeable tiredness that comes on suddenly and often comes and goes or never stops. This condition has become a source of mystery and there are no conclusive authorities who agree on exactly what it is, but many of us experience bouts of fatigue when we just can't find the energy to get on with our daily life. This stretch of chronic fatigue may have been brought on by a period of intense stress, perhaps the death of someone close to you, losing a job or the end of a relationship, but it may be that you have no idea why you feel so low, you just do!

Chronic fatigue is described by SupportME as a "major depressive illness with psychotic or melancholic features." Depression and chronic fatigue are inextricably linked but it is not known which one causes which fallout. However, it might be that a lack of physical and mental energy in the body, caused by nutritional deficiency combined with overuse of processed foods, causes a long-lasting fatigue. It could be the right time, therefore, to look at some diet changes and, in particular, some foods that help fight fatigue.

Here are some recommendations to help give you vitality and energy:

* **Eat a large breakfast.** When we wake up our brain needs fuel. A good breakfast improves alertness and concentration, helps shed pounds by preventing overeating during the day and prevents obesity, diabetes and heart disease. A good breakfast refills our energy stores, keeping lethargy at bay during the morning hours. Oats are a particularly encouraging breakfast to fight fatigue as they are a low-GI food, which helps balance the blood sugar and prevents the highs and lows that get us grabbing high-sugar/fat foods.
Fatigue-busting food: oats, muesli, fruit smoothies.
* **Eat plenty of fruit and vegetables.** These are packed with vitamins and minerals that you need to keep your immune system strong and energy levels high, hence eating fruit for snacks between meals is a good way to get a zing.
Fatigue-busting food: apples, bananas, papaya.
* **Eat foods rich in iron.** Iron enables blood to carry oxygen to the body's organs. Deprived of adequate oxygen, the brain cannot function optimally, leading to lack of mental agility and feelings of fatigue.
Fatigue-busting food: garbanzo beans, kidney beans, prunes.
* **Eat protein.** Protein contains the amino acid tryptophan, precursor of serotonin, a neurotransmitter that promotes a calm, relaxed feeling and which helps to fight emotional fatigue. Protein-rich foods also contain tyrosine, a precursor to the neurotransmitter dopamine, which is a promoter of alertness, attention, and motivation.
Fatigue-busting food: fish, soybeans, peanuts.

✳ **Eat some raw foods.** Raw foods have vast quantities of enzymes, which will help perk up a sluggish digestion and raise your energy levels.
Fatigue-busting food: carrots, apples, celery.

✳ **Drink plenty of water.** Dehydration leads to drowsiness which also makes you feel irritable.

Finally, don't get too hungry, as your blood sugar could fall, leaving you feeling listless and dull. Smaller meals also help to keep insulin levels constant, avoiding fluctuations of energy and mood.

2. DEPRESSION

Diet plays a huge part in the way our mood is regulated and this is what this whole book is about. However, as depression is such a high "food sensitive" mood, we will look at some immediate ways to feel better through food.

On the whole, there are two sides to the way we can manage depression with our food: by looking at the foods which exacerbate depression—what to cut out; and by looking at the foods which alleviate depression—what to get in. In other words, it's about getting out the junk and getting good food in—a two-pronged attack.

What to cut out

When we look at the foods that cause depression, there is no doubt that a high-fat/salt/sugar diet is going to badly affect your mood. All five of the bad-mood foods sections of this chapter explain how they affect your mood and argue that a modern diet of processed foods contributes to the body feeling lethargic, stressed and depressed. However, if there is one main culprit, it would be sugar.

The reason sugar has such a negative impact on depression is that sugar causes a rise in the insulin levels of the blood.

This also raises the serotonin level, a natural mood lifter, in the brain. These sugars cause the body to have an artificial, chemical, mental high, resulting in a lift in mood. Continuous large doses of sugar over a long time usually cause the brain's serotonin production to slow or shut down. When the body cuts back on serotonin production it reduces the amount of serotonin available in the body at any given time. The lack of enough serotonin in the brain causes depression.

If an individual is a high sugar eater, to maintain a normal level of serotonin in the brain the individual must eat more and more sugar to avoid the feeling of depression and maintain a normal mood. This causes the swinging cycle of the "sugar high / sugar low" and the body then needs more sugar to feel "normal." In many ways, this cycle is similar to alcohol dependency, when the alcoholic needs more and more alcohol to realize the same effect that the alcohol once had; conversely, the more alcohol that is consumed, the more the body tolerates it and so increasing the need for higher consumption.

Continuously high levels of sugar create an artificial energy which we become used to and may have always felt. It is hard to escape sugar as even powdered baby milk contains sugar and this will give us the taste of it from a very early age. However, the craving for sugar is beatable, and within three days you may notice a profound difference in your mood and your craving as you turn to other foods.

> Did you know that dried dates can cut a sugar craving down dead? Eat them before you expect a sugar hunger.

What to get in

Tryptophan – Foods rich in the amino acid, tryptophan, facilitate the body's uptake of the wonderful neurotransmitter, serotonin. We want plenty of serotonin to feel good and beat depression. High tryptophan foods are:

✳ Soy products: soy milk, tofu, soybean nuts
✳ Seafood
✳ Turkey
✳ Whole grains
✳ Beans
✳ Rice
✳ Houmous
✳ Lentils
✳ Hazelnuts, peanuts
✳ Eggs
✳ Sesame seeds, sunflower seeds

Omega-3: Omega-3 is another compound that is brilliant for fighting depression. This is covered extensively in the next chapter, as it is one of the Superfoods (see "Fish Food"), and has been proven to lift depression. Suffice it to say that this important nutrient is critical for good health. Omega-3 fatty acids are a form of polyunsaturated fats, one of four basic types of fat that the body derives from food. All polyunsaturated fats, including the omega-3s, are increasingly recognized as important to human health, but they cannot be produced by the body, which means they need to be added to our diet. A lack of omega-3 mood-boosting nutrients may lead to depression and other mental health problems. Interestingly, the oil used to help the child with a degenerative nerve disorder in the popular film *Lorenzo's Oil* was an omega-3 fatty acid.

Here is a list of the gorgeous omega-3 fat sources:
✳ Fish (covered extensively in Fish Food, Chapter 5)
✳ Canola oil
✳ Olive oil
✳ Flaxseed oil
✳ Walnuts
✳ Venison

Folic Acid: Folic acid is also a brilliant depression fighter and research shows that people with low levels of folic acid are more likely to suffer from depression—scientists at the American Psychiatric Association recommend plenty of folic acid daily as a preventative measure for depression. Folic acid is a water-soluble vitamin and the body can't retain it for long, with any excess being expelled in the urine. This means that any of us could be deficient in folic acid at any one time; it is a hard vitamin to keep in the body. Eating some of these foods will help keep your levels high:

* Beetroot
* Spinach
* Broccoli
* Avocados
* Asparagus
* Dried beans
* Soy products
* Brussels sprouts

3. LACKLUSTER SKIN

Do you long for great skin but, no matter how much you spend on costly cosmetics, you just can't seem to get the results you're looking for? We all have those days when we look in the mirror and our skin says it all! A few days on the trot where we've worked our socks off and grabbed food on the go, or when we have been partying nonstop and have neglected ourselves; it will begin to show in our skin. When we suffer depression we can neglect ourselves nutritionally, and this can show up in lackluster skin. Then we look in the mirror and it reflects back someone who is not on top of life, which can quickly send us into a spiral of despair. Added to that, if we are insecure about our looks, it doesn't take much in the way of a "bad skin day" to make us feel worse.

In spite of this, lackluster skin has more to do with our diet than the type of skin products we use, which is great news for those of us who are looking for ways to get better-looking skin without forking out a fortune for expensive skin-care products. Skin is the largest organ in our body and, as we know, our organs need optimum nutrition to stay healthy—so if you feed your body vitality through your food, your skin will glow with radiance. It really is possible to eat your way to great skin and you don't have to change your whole life. There are three areas to concentrate on which will get your skin on the road to recovery.

Ditch the high-GI carbohydrates

Foods high in refined carbohydrates are called high-GI carbohydrates and these can cause a hormonal surge that produces excess sebum in the body. Sebum is the fatty substance excreted by the sebaceous glands in the skin. It is necessary because our skin needs a certain amount of lubrication, but if your sebaceous glands produce too much sebum, they tend to get blocked (blackheads) and infected (acne). Low-GI carbohydrates, on the other hand, contain certain types of carbohydrates that are broken down slowly by the digestive system, which result in a gradual release of glucose into the bloodstream. This has less of an impact on blood-sugar levels and may help control excess sebum.

Here is a quick list of high- and low-GI carbohydrates:

High-GI carbohydrates — lackluster skin foods	Low-GI carbohydrates — great skin foods
White bread	Wholemeal bread
White pasta	Whole-grain pasta
White rice	Brown rice
Refined breakfast cereal	Oats

Up the anti

Your skin is designed to provide a natural protective barrier to the sun; but it needs help. Studies show that the worst thing for your skin is sun damage. Even in our gray winters, the sun can be detrimental to your skin and it needs all the help it can get. A good nutritional defense plan is one way to help you to better skin and there is no better nutrition than antioxidants. They help in slowing down the ageing of skin and are probably the most important ingredient in foods to help fight free-radical damage, which is thought to be the biggest cause of premature ageing. Antioxidants are found in abundance in densely colored fruit and vegetables, the darker and denser the color, the better. Eat at least five portions of fruit and vegetables a day. Here are some of the highest ranking antioxidant foods:

* Cranberries
* Blueberries
* Blackberries
* Pinto, kidney and black beans
* Artichokes
* Prunes
* Raspberries
* Red apples

Vitamin C

Vitamin C offers outstanding protection against the oxidative stress that is believed to be a major factor in the ageing process. It is particularly valuable in our skin because of the often extreme oxidative stress caused by the sun and because of the powerful antioxidants of this wonderful vitamin. Furthermore, one of vitamin C's most important functions in our skin (and throughout the entire body) is to regenerate the molecules of vitamin E. After it has helped to neutralize free radical, Vitamin E can be recycled to act as an antioxidant over and over again, making its use by the body far more efficient than it would be otherwise, and making our daily requirement for it much less.

Eat plenty of the following:
* Citrus fruits or berries
* Dried fruit, especially apricots and figs
* Spinach, broccoli
* A handful of almonds, hazelnuts or sunflower seeds

4. INSOMNIA

Sleep deprivation is a major cause of depression. An estimated 25 percent of adults suffer from insomnia and approximately 18 million prescriptions are written every year for sleeping pills. Sleep loss can result in high blood levels of glucose, which can be the source of memory loss, irritability and depression. For some people, their whole life is ruled by how much sleep they get or don't get and this can play a critical part in their whole wellbeing. Diet can play a large part in helping us to get a good night's sleep. Again, we need to take the two-pronged attack: what to ditch and what to eat.

What to ditch to prevent insomnia
* **Coffee and tea.** Don't drink within four hours of before going to bed. Caffeine is a great stimulant for the nervous system because it enters the bloodstream fifteen minutes after it has been consumed and it takes the body six hours to eliminate half of it.
* **Alcohol.** Although alcohol helps you to initially feel sleepy, it can keep you from getting deep sleep, which may mean a less restful night's sleep. Alcohol causes the release of adrenaline so, when the drink wears off, you may wake up feeling tired. We've all had those mornings after the night before!
* **Sodas.** These may contain caffeine, but also the sugar content will make your digestion work overtime and therefore disturb your sleep. Plus, a full bladder will wake you up.

✳ Chocolate. Because of the high sugar and fat content in most chocolate that we buy, the digestive system will be busy trying to digest it and this will keep you up. Added to this, chocolate is a stimulant which will keep your heart rate up and you want your heart rate to be as low as possible for a good night's sleep.

✳ Spicy foods. Sleeplessness has also been associated with spicy foods. Excess intake of spices can result in heartburn that gets aggravated once you lie down. As a result you may find sleeping a problem. Moreover, heartburn can also awaken you in the middle of the night.

Food to eat to promote a good sleep

✳ Foods that contain tryptophan may have some benefit in promoting sleepiness. As discussed under "Depression," this amino acid is also central to all normal brain functions, of which sleep patterns are included.

✳ Replace highly spiced foods with gentle foods such as lettuce. Lettuce has an opium-related substance with traces of anti-cramping agents. Lettuce should be an integral part of your evening diet if you are suffering from insomnia.

✳ A salad and pasta meal is really good for promoting sleep because pasta is high in complex carbohydrates, which increase serotonin and will give you a mild sleepy feeling, and salad contains lettuce.

✳ Replace coffee and tea with herbal or fruit teas.

✳ Bananas are a good dessert and, because it is a tryptophan-rich food, it will boost your melatonin, the hormone that aids sleep.

5. LOSS OF LIBIDO

There is no single answer to what constitutes loss of libido and the reasons will depend on the individual and their very personal circumstances. Losing our libido, however, can be a trigger for depression in itself, because when we lose our libido we lose one of the primeval driving forces that helps to shape us as individuals. From the other side, in diagnosed depression, loss of libido is a symptom in almost 70 percent of cases. If the doctor then prescribes you an antidepressant, the chances are that your libido could take a further dive, because loss of libido is one of the side effects of antidepressants.

One thing is known, stress is a top sex zapper. A constant state of stress and anxiety is also a trigger for depression and fatigue. These conditions are not conducive to having a high sexual libido. Generally speaking, men seem to become more stressed about work and their work performance; also, general ill health, drinking quantities of alcohol or being overweight may explain a low sex drive in men. Women, on the other hand, become stressed about other issues. As more women are going out to work, they are finding that all their responsibilities, but particularly their domestic responsibilities, are making them feel overloaded and stressed. Other stress factors for women are: conflict within a relationship, weight gain, post-childbirth, the onset of menopause, or hormonal imbalances. It tends to be a roundabout because you may be stressed and turn to the bad mood foods for comfort. Then you feel lethargic, depressed and dumpy—then feel less attractive, so further decrease sexual desire.

The mind is willing – but is the body?

Don't always assume that lack of desire is only psychological. Having loads of natural energy and vitality may be as important in rekindling a flagging libido as a "talking therapy." Nutritional deficiencies can adversely affect your hormone levels and sexual organs. By eating to revive a sex drive you may be pleasantly surprised at the results. If you felt a hundred percent healthy, happy and in love with your body, they may have to hold you back on the sex front!

Getting started on the 7-Day Food Plan for stress is a brilliant way to start turning your libido misfortunes around.

By eating a diet that includes plenty of low-GI foods, such as butter beans, kidney beans, garbanzo beans, etc., you may begin to feel more energy; mix that with a decrease in sugar and refined carbohydrates, your energy levels will begin to balance and you will feel better for longer.

By ensuring you get the five portions of fresh fruit and vegetables a day, you will be eating more fiber, which will help you to feel "lighter," together with lots of aphrodisiac enzymes. And you know what they say about oats! What oats do is to give a slow release of energy over a longer period of time. This will help to avoid the 11 a.m. "low" when you have to grab a quick sugar snack to keep going. If you choose the oats in the breakfast menu from one of the 7-Day Food Plans, together with an overall well-balanced diet, you could feel the difference in your morning energy.

Oysters—the romance food? There is no research to back up this legendary aphrodisiac claim but there are some benefits to be had from eating oysters. In fact, seafood generally contains trace elements of zinc, iodine and iron—all necessary to utilize the energy in your food.

And finally, we are hearing about the powerful and sexy properties of raw sauerkraut, which is a pickled cabbage. There are no scientific studies to back up these claims, but more and more people are talking about the great sexy mood booster that this vegetable has given them. It's worth a look!

6. PREMENSTRUAL TENSION

Premenstrual tension can be a fiend. Some women have a little discomfort for a day or two before a period, but for many women PMT can bring about a week or even two weeks of emotional chaos and physical misery. If you suffer from depression, bad PMT can do nothing but exacerbate the symptoms as other factors come into play like extreme fatigue, volatile mood swings and a tense, aching body.

As with all other bad-food fallouts, eating bad-mood food can be up to 75 percent of the problem and may aggravate PMT. It is an easy solution to dive into "comfort foods" consisting of high levels of salt, fat and sugar at this time of the month. Statements such as "pamper yourself" or "take some time out for you" can feel condescending and don't get to the essence of PMT, making us feel even more irritated and snappy.

However, there are answers in the diet, and this is so exciting because bad PMT can be a thing of the past with a few changes in what we eat! Here are some dietary ways to help overcome the misery of PMT.

Fluids

One of the main problems of PMT is fluid retention. Fluid retention is very common and it might make you feel fuzzy or emotionally sensitive, where little things become major frustrations. You may suffer from lackluster skin, have no energy, your muscles ache and you feel tense and stressed. Contrary to popular belief, fluid retention is not caused by drinking too much fluid but due to hormone levels, too much salt or too little exercise. Often the body retains fluid because we don't drink enough. It's easy to mistake dehydration for hunger and eat when we need water. But, water also helps digestion and elimination whereas dehydration can cause headaches, fatigue and constipation. It's also great for your skin.

So the answer is to up your fluid intake: increase your water drinking to six glasses a day. You can also eat natural liquorice to help you get relief from fluid retention.

Omega-3

What more can we say? These powerful nutrients are here again as a wonder aid for our bodies. Omega-3s help the hormonal system to function properly, producing prostaglandins, which help to produce progesterone, and which helps prevent PMT and associated pain with the monthly cycle, heavy bleeding and menopausal symptoms. It is best found in oily fish and cold-pressed oils. It has also been found to help tremendously with some hormonal problems like inflammation, weight issues, blood pressure, blood sugar and high cholesterol.

Good omega-3 sources include: oily fish, almonds, sesame, sunflower and pumpkin seeds and their oil, avocados, linseed and hemp seeds and their oils.

Magnesium

Magnesium deficiency has been strongly linked to PMT symptoms. It is necessary for the absorption of calcium and is the primary mineral required by the adrenal glands to help the body cope with stress. Increasing your magnesium levels could help with muscle cramps, sleep problems, fatigue and depression.

Good magnesium foods include: spinach, avocados, barley, pumpkin and sunflower seeds, Brazil nuts, buckwheat and almonds.

B6

Vitamin B6 is excellent for keeping PMT symptoms at bay. It increases the build-up of magnesium within the cells of the body. When balanced with foods high in magnesium, foods containing B6 can reduce susceptibility to mood changes during the menstrual cycle. B6 is also a mood enhancer, excellent for irritability, aids good sleep and helps alleviate depression.

Good B6 foods include: sweet potatoes, whole grains, tofu, nuts, seeds, pulses, avocados, apricots and asparagus.

7. MIGRAINE

If you are run down, stressed and depressed, you may be at a higher risk of migraine. Migraines are severe, pounding headaches so intense and overwhelming that they can be unbearable. Migraine attacks may last from a few minutes or up to several days and can be completely debilitating. You may know if a migraine is coming on by a temporary loss of peripheral vision or by seeing wavy lines. Once the migraine starts you may suffer a throbbing, pulsating pain, nausea and/or vomiting, loss of appetite or a painful aversion to light.

The exact underlying cause of migraines isn't known. The current thinking suggests that migraines are the result of spasms in the arteries, which supply blood to the brain, as a result of constriction. This is then thought to cause other arteries in the brain to rapidly dilate, which triggers the release of chemicals that cause intense pain and inflammation. Migraines may be brought on by stress, overwork, extreme weather change, prescribed drug use or hormonal changes.

Bad migraine foods

Foods that bring on migraines could be associated with fluctuations in sugar levels and may include particular foods that contain compounds known as amines, which are associated with smoked or cured meats such as bacon and hot dogs. Foods containing the amine tyramine, like red wine and blue cheeses, are also said to bring on migraines. Peanut butter, yogurt, sour cream, onions, pickles, freshly baked yeast products, alcohol and coffee have all been linked to migraine attacks.

Change your basic diet

Again, as with all the "bad-food fallouts," making some changes in your overall diet will help to play a large part in making your body feel better, with more energy and a good-mood boost. The foods that appear to have the most detrimental effect on those people who suffer from migraines are processed foods and foods not in their natural state. It would seem reasonable that eating wholesome foods could go a long way to tackling migraines, and any one of the 7-Day Food Plans could be of great benefit to those who suffer.

The 80/20 rule

The 80/20 rule is an idea that is used by many people who work in the medical and complementary health field. This rule has been adapted from the original concept conceived by an Italian economist Vilfredo Pareto in 1906. It was a mathematical formula to describe the unequal distribution of wealth in his country, observing that 20 percent of the people owned 80 percent of the wealth. But the numbers work surprisingly well for many other areas, including the 80/20 food rule, which means that if you aim to eat good, wholesome food 80 percent of the time, you can then afford to eat the more high-fat/sugar/salt foods the rest of the time—it can be a very simple but effective way of helping you to manage your diet if you are prone to eating processed foods and are finding it difficult to cut them out altogether.

Omega-3

If there is one food that is thought to help migraine sufferers it is omega-3 fatty acids. Again this magical nutrient comes to the forefront as a powerful tonic and, because it is a "brain food," it would seem logical that it could help those suffering from migraines.

A study in Sweden in 1995 showed that people who ate 2.4g of omega-3 fatty acids every day reported their migraine attacks reduced by 60 percent. This amount of omega-3 is found in a small can of sardines in tomato sauce. A sardine snack may be just what you need to help you beat migraines.

Riboflavin

Riboflavin, otherwise known as Vitamin B2, is needed by all cells to make the energy to carry out daily activities. Studies have shown that riboflavin is a great benefit to migraine sufferers. The improvement seen in migraine sufferers is up to 50 percent, sometimes even working as well as prescription drugs at reducing the frequency of attacks. And there are no bad side effects associated with riboflavin compared to these drugs. Expect to see results after two to three months of increasing your intake of riboflavin. Good sources of riboflavin include calf's liver, spent (a type of grain), spinach, soy nuts and almonds.

Magnesium

Magnesium is an essential mineral and is very similar to riboflavin, in that it is needed by cells for proper energy metabolism. Low magnesium levels may therefore make people more prone to attacks through defects in cell metabolism. It also helps with the normal function of blood vessels. Low levels of magnesium seem to make the blood vessels in the head more susceptible to migraine triggers. As many as 50 percent of migraine sufferers have low levels of magnesium in their brains or in their blood. Getting more magnesium may significantly reduce the frequency of migraine attacks. By increasing both riboflavin and magnesium, there could be a good chance that your migraines will subside, and this is a positive step toward feeling better in yourself and then being able to concentrate on fighting depression with other good-mood foods. Good magnesium foods include raw peanuts, tofu, chard and broccoli.

8. IRRITABILITY

A classic sign of depression is irritability—feeling unhappy, behaving with snappiness, fed-up-ness or petulance. Irritability is usually described as "a sign that a child is coming down with an illness" and indeed that is a perfect description of irritability. When you feel irritable and fed up, it is perfectly possible to feel like a child on the edge of something else; for many, irritability is a frustration when things just don't go your way.

On an emotional level, irritability can be a sure sign of buried anger, and nipping at others or stamping feet is a way of letting the anger seep out a little without having to deal with it head on. In effect it's acting as a pressure cooker by letting a little heat out of the system. However, if it isn't dealt with as a whole, and the pressure cooker becomes overheated, the whole pot could explode. Buried anger leads to depression and looking at anger and its manifestations can go a long way to getting a handle on irritability as well as depression. For a guide to managing your anger see my first book, *Beat Depression and Reclaim Your Life.*

From a food point of view, one of the reasons for irritability can be a lack of fiber. It would make sense, because fiber helps eliminate waste from the body and acts as an internal cleaning brush. So, if you are physically blocked you may become emotionally blocked. Conversely, if you are emotionally blocked, you will be tenser and this tension advances to the internal organs where the tension will stiffen and inhibit their effectiveness, so your digestive system may slow down. By relaxing your stomach muscles you will free some tension and allow your digestion a little breathing space.

Foodwise, the best thing you can do is start the day with breakfast. Skipping breakfast can cause irritability and fatigue which can also cause a slump in blood sugar and will cause you to feel a lot more irritable and depressed.

Good breakfast ideas are in the start of the 7-Day Food Plans on page 165.

9. SEASONAL AFFECTIVE DISORDER (SAD)

With the onset of winter and the days getting shorter, people with SAD often feel depressed and tired. That point at which the clocks turn back in the fall can be the beginning of a long and dark time if you suffer from SAD. If you suffer from depression as well, this can be the worst time of year, with the extra hour of darkness each evening rendering you even more tired and depressed during the long winter months.

There is certainly a lot of ambiguity surrounding SAD. No one is sure precisely what causes it. What is known is that sufferers may gain weight because they crave carbohydrates or sugary foods, and this can perpetuate other food-related problems such as fatigue and a general feeling of poor health. They may become socially withdrawn or irritable, and are unable to concentrate, which all add up to a depressive state.

There is a possible link of SAD with the production of a hormone called melatonin, which the body produces more of in darkness. It makes people become drowsy, and it is thought that people with SAD release more melatonin than others. Melatonin is produced by the brain and made from the amino acid tryptophan. This hormone is known to play a role in regulating the body-clock's natural wake-sleep cycle. Melatonin levels increase as exposure to light decreases and this is why, if you suffer from SAD, it occurs in the winter.

It would make sense that the body would respond in this way because it simply wants us to get more sleep when there's less light about. However, this body-clock doesn't appear to fit in with our modern life and in trying to fight it we may inadvertently render ourselves depressed.

Eat well

Because SAD sufferers tend to crave junk food, it becomes a vicious cycle: feel tired—hit the high-fat/salt/sugar foods—feel bad—get a "what the hell" approach to diet—eat more junk—feel worse. By following the 7-Day Food Plan for chronic fatigue on page 195, you will begin to notice the results within 24 hours as you start to get high-energy foods into your system, which will start to knock the bad-food fallout cycle on the head.

Get light

One route to fighting SAD is to ensure the body gets lots of light. As obvious as this may sound, taking lots of walks in the winter can help to do this as well lifting the spirits. Exercise has also been discovered to be an effective treatment for depression.

Vitamin D

It's called the sunlight vitamin, because the body produces it when the sun's ultraviolet B (UVB) rays strike the skin. It is the only vitamin the body manufactures naturally and is technically considered a hormone. Vitamin D has been a key nutrient to help SAD sufferers and one study found that people with SAD who received increased amounts of Vitamin D undertook a significant improvement in depression symptoms after one month. Foods high in vitamin D include prawns, milk, cod, eggs.

10. POOR MEMORY

One of the classic signs of depression is poor memory. It is significant that in times of despair or trauma the brain refuses to recall memories, because some of those memories may be painful and the psyche just doesn't want to remember them. Poor memory may also be impaired by stress. Stressed-out people tend to lack concentration and attention and can suffer from a mild attention deficiency disorder.

Depressed people generally have decreased levels of serotonin, and as serotonin helps the brain carry messages it may explain the reduced brain-cell activity. Additionally serotonin helps regulate arousal and interest or stimulation in normal activities and let's face it, if you're not interested in your work, relationships or life in general, the need to keep your memory sharp loses its appeal. So by following the 7-Day Food Plan for depression and boosting the wonderful serotonin hormone, you will automatically increase your memory capability.

Manganese

Manganese is one of those little-heard-of nutrients that the body cannot do without. It is an essential mineral necessary for good health and, particularly, good brain function. It aids wellbeing by helping oxygen transfer from the lungs to the cells, and oxygenated cells are just what the body needs for a good memory. Symptoms of manganese deficiencies include nerve and hearing problems, lack of concentration and mental confusion, all of which are connected to depression, stress and poor memory. By targeting these bad-food fallout symptoms we can help fight depression and its respective cousins. Raw nuts and seeds, wholewheat pasta, oats, pineapple and whole grains are all good sources of manganese.

5

SUPERFOODS TO FIGHT DEPRESSION, FATIGUE AND STRESS

Sometimes the mere act of eating can make us happy, but there is a growing body of evidence suggesting that eating the right foods can help us beat depression. There's a whole array of great foods that will help you improve your health, but which ones are specifically good for fighting depression? This chapter presents the top ten best foods that can work with your body to support and lift the mood, offer an energy pick-up or soothe stressed nerves.

1. FISH FOOD

During the 1970s scientists made the first associations between omega-3 fats and human health, whilst studying the Eskimos of Greenland. They noticed that this group of people suffered far less from certain diseases than their European friends and that their diet was rich in fats from eating whale, seal, and salmon. The researchers finally realized that it was the type of fats they were eating, omega-3s, that provided the real health benefits. During their studies they noted that the rate of depression in this type of people was way below the standard rates of depression in the West.

Then, in 1999, a landmark study was undertaken at Harvard University on people suffering depression. Half the group was given omega-3 oils and the other half was given a placebo. The study was due to go on for nine months but was halted after four months due to its outstanding results with the omega-3 group saying their depression had significantly decreased. Many other such studies have highlighted the effectiveness of omega-3s on depression, so much so that some patients have been able to come off their antidepressant drugs because they have found themselves free of the depressive symptoms from which they used to suffer.

The impression we get is that this discovery is new, but history tells us that our ancestors used to acquire an abundant supply of omega-3 fat through their diets which were rich in fish and also game like venison and wild fowl. These animals have a much higher amount of omega-3 fats than farm-raised animals because wild game eat a lot of green grass and vegetables. Today our main source of meat comes from animals that are intensively raised on farms and are fed a diet rich in processed grains, which are low in omega-3 fats. As consumption of omega-3 fatty acids has reduced from the Western food supply, the rates of depression have dramatically increased in Western countries. I do not believe that these figures can be explained by changes in social structures only and it is perhaps the declining amounts of omega-3s that we ingest that has had an influence on the increasing rates of depression.

Our bodies need omega-3 fats for several reasons. They are the key to healthy arteries, a strong heart and keeping the immune system healthy, but one of their most significant roles may be in the brain. Although the way in which these fats work is unproven, it is thought that perhaps the omega-3s feed the brain, which makes the membranes more resilient and therefore eases the flow of the neurotransmitters. It would make sense when you realize that 70 percent of the brain's membranes are made up of fatty-acid molecules, so when you eat omega-3s you are feeding your brain a similar component to its derivation.

Omega-3 fatty acids may also chemically influence major depression. Certain chemicals in the brain, called cytokines, which play a role in the inflammation response, also cause feelings of depression. Omega-3 fatty acids, and EPA in particular, block the action of these cytokines. Incidentally, this is also how some antidepressants work. Added to that, omega-3s have a direct effect on the levels of serotonin in the body and if you don't have enough serotonin, you're more likely to be depressed.

Although it is possible to get omega-3 fats from some plants, with flaxseed being the number one provider, the type of fat that helps depression is the "long chain" omega-3. This term refers to the chemical structure of the omega-3 and is only found in fish. The type of omega-3 found in plants is called the "short chain" variety and, although it is good for general health, it is the long-chain omega-3 which is more potent to help beat depression. These fats have to be found solely in our diet because they cannot be produced by the body. The types of fish to eat are oil-rich fish such as salmon, herring, mackerel, trout, tuna and sardines.

Just two portions of oily fish a week can help you to beat depression. Here are two delicious recipes that can give you a portion of oily fish and get you started on beating the blues.

BLISSFUL MACKEREL PÂTÉ

A simple but delicious pâté put together in just five minutes. This is perfect for a quick lunch.

(Serves 2)
1 can (4-oz.) mackerel fillets in olive oil
1 teaspoon bottled capers, rinsed and roughly chopped
1/4 cup chopped fresh flat-leaf parsley
1 medium ripe avocado, peeled, seeded, and chopped
2 tablespoons plain yogurt
Juice of 1/2 lemon
Other half of the lemon to garnish

Method: Place all the ingredients into a mixing bowl, making sure you flake the fish gently. Mix and serve with wholewheat toast and a quarter of the lemon to squeeze over.

HAPPY HERRINGS WITH OATS

(Serves 2)

4 medium herring fillets

1/3 cup coarse steel-cut oats

2 tablespoons olive oil

2 ounces raw chorizo sausage

1 lemon, quartered to garnish

Fresh green salad to serve

Method: Roll the herring fillets in the oats. Heat the oil in a skillet. Slice the chorizo into 1/4-inch slices and fry in the skillet until crisp; remove from the pan and keep warm.

Place the herrings in the pan and fry them in the same oil until the oats turn golden brown. Place the chorizo and herrings onto a plate. Garnish with the lemon for squeezing over and serve with a salad.

2. BEAT THE BLUES WITH BERRIES

Berries are a commanding source of mood-boosting products, and the genius of their make-up and what they have to offer those who suffer from depression, stress or fatigue is why berries are a superfood. They are crammed with disease-fighting phytochemicals and just a handful of berries a day can help you jump-start your way to feeling better. Some of the most potent phytochemicals are antioxidants. We need a good source of antioxidants to keep our cells healthy, and especially if we are depressed or suffer chronic fatigue, so that they will support our immune system. The direct link between emotional and physical health was established in 2003 with a breakthrough study at the US National Academy of Sciences. Researchers discovered that the happier the volunteers were, the stronger their immune system was.

How antioxidants work

To better explain how antioxidants work, cut an organic apple and an organic lemon in half. Squeeze the juice of the lemon over one half of the apple on the exposed side but leave the other half as it is. Leave both halves for thirty minutes. When you go back and check the condition of the two halves, you will see that the untreated half has gone brown and has started to dry out. This is a free-radical attack and is caused by oxidization. Rusting is another form of oxidization and happens when iron gets left lying around in damp conditions and iron, water and oxygen mix together. This weakens the metal, eventually destroying it. It is this same type of corrosion that occurs to our cells, and we need antioxidants to stop the corrosion. Antioxidants counteract these oxygen free radicals, and bind with them before they can cause damage. And what makes berries so interesting is that they contain an astonishing concentration of antioxidants in relation to their size.

Blueberries

Blueberries are the number one superfood of all the berries. Though tiny in size, their age-defying antioxidants have been linked with boosts in memory and eyesight. For example, 4 ounces of blueberries delivers as much antioxidant strength as five servings of other fruits and vegetables. This density of antioxidants in the blueberry has recently been hailed as a breakthrough for degenerative diseases like Alzheimer's and senile dementia. It's the anti-ageing function that is so effective for depression, because fatigue can make you feel so old and being depressed can make you feel so debilitated.

Depression is part of the ageing process and the older we get, the more likely we are to suffer with depression and chronic anxiety, so munching on a handful of blueberries instead of reaching into the cookie jar is one way to give our body the goodness of this powerful berry. A substantial amount of the antioxidant is to be found in the skin of the blueberry, so when you buy blueberry juice, make sure you get a product that contains lots of sediment at the bottom, because this is where the goodness can be found. As we are more at risk of cancer if we are depressed, because we tend to eat more processed food, we need to increase foods which offer a natural protection.

Lower cholesterol – lower depression

The blueberry is also loaded with pectin fiber, which helps to lower cholesterol levels. In fact, research shows that a compound in blueberries acts just as effectively as drugs to reduce levels of bad cholesterol in mice, but without the negative side effects (e.g. muscle wasting) of prescribed drugs. Having high cholesterol puts you in a higher risk of heart disease and the risk of heart disease is doubled in people with depression, so eat your way out of the high-risk group and incorporate a good dose of antioxidants in your diet.

So, if you want to do one simple thing for your health, add a handful of blueberries to your diet.

Strawberries

Since Roman times, strawberries were reputed to have therapeutic powers for healing bad gums and digestive problems. But now strawberries are getting some of the credence they deserve. To begin with, they are packed with vitamin C, which is said to check the accumulation of carcinogenic compounds in the intestine and to protect the good cholesterol from destruction by oxygen free radicals due to their antioxidant properties. They contain plenty of potassium (good for lowering blood pressure), are known to fight heart disease and contain pectin (a cholesterol-reducing fiber), which is a powerful antidote to stress and anxiety. They also provide a number of vitamins and minerals that support overall human health. They are high in fiber, folic acid, potassium and manganese.

Cranberries

Cranberries are perhaps best known for preventing urinary-tract infections, which are more common in people who are stressed and run down, and science is beginning to suggest that there could be some truth in this old folklore. Cranberries contain proanthocyanidins, which are the compounds believed responsible for the anti-stick mechanism that helps maintain urinary-tract health. In other words, proanthocyanidins "disable" certain harmful bacteria in the body, so the bacteria don't stick to the walls of the urinary tract. Urinary disorders are particularly prevalent in women whose immune systems are low, which may be caused by depression.

An amazing treatment for the stress ulcer

Cranberries have also been shown to help patients with ulcers, which are more common in people who suffer from stress. Prolonged stress lowers the immune system, leaving the body more open to infection and particularly infection by the Helicobacter pylori bacteria to which ulcers are increasingly being attributed. Cranberries have been shown to inhibit the adhesion of these bacteria to human gastric mucus in the stomach, helping to prevent ulcers.

Fatigue fighter

A further attribute of the fabulous cranberry is the significant amount of flavonoids and polyphenolic compounds that it contains, suggesting that cranberries may offer a natural defence against "bad cholesterol," which results in restricted blood flow within the arteries. As blood flow decreases, the chances of suffering angina, a thrombosis or heart attack increase. These conditions contribute to a sense of depression, because the oxygen in our bodies is depleted and we feel a sense of fatigue.

If you are looking for the benefits of cranberries to help improve your urinary health, don't drink the carton juice from the supermarket, which can contain sugar, additives and preservatives. Instead eat fresh cranberries from the refrigerator section or grab a bag of dried cranberries from the baking section to give you a perfect snack in between your meals.

Raspberries

Raspberries are the princess of the berry world; delicate, exquisite and incredibly exotic. A punnet of raspberries makes a sumptuous dessert and really doesn't need much in the way of dressing. But the reason we should include them as much as possible once their season is in full swing is that they are known for their ability to fight cancer thanks to their phytochemical content and abundant supply of vitamins and minerals. These all contribute to our overall sense of wellbeing and, as a result, help us to feel physically and emotionally better.

Berries – healthy and versatile

You can mix berries with yogurt, sprinkle them onto breakfast cereal or eat as a snack straight out of the bowl. If fresh berries are unavailable, eat them dried or frozen. Our berry season is generally from May to September, and if you pick your own at a farm shop or pick blackberries from the brambles, you can easily freeze them for use at a later date. Simply place them on a tray and place in your freezer. Eat a handful a day to get the fabulous benefits they have to offer. If you have frozen the berries, adding them to a smoothie directly from the freezer chills the smoothie and gives it a luxurious taste that is impossible to resist.

SMOOTHIE BOOSTER

If you need a boost to start your day, look no farther than this recipe for a "wake-me-up" smoothie. You can put any type of fruit in with your berries but this recipe includes apples and pears, as they are easily available and great for the digestive system.

(Serves 1)
1 apple, quartered and cored
1 pear, quartered and cored
Handful of berries — fresh, frozen, or dried
A splash of fruit juice
Fruit yogurt to taste

Method: Blend all the ingredients until smooth, then drink straightaway. Your insides will feel like they've had a wake-up call.

MOUTH-WATERING BERRY PUDDING

This is the simplest but most sophisticated way of eating summer berries to end a meal. It's elegant enough for a dinner party and healthy enough to eat without any guilt.

(Serves 4)
2 punnets of strawberries
2 punnets of raspberries
4 tablespoons water or kirsch (or your favorite liqueur)
2 teaspoons unpasteurized honey
Greek-style or thick plain yogurt to serve

Method: Rinse and hull the strawberries and place in a serving bowl. Rinse the raspberries and place them in a saucepan with the water or liqueur and simmer until soft; set aside to cool. When cool, stir in the honey and purée in a blender or food processor until smooth. Pour over the strawberries and serve with yogurt for spooning over the top.

FRESH BERRY GELATIN

This recipe is a fun and nourishing way of eating berries that all the family will enjoy. You can leave it to set in stylish wine glasses for a dinner party, or put it in an old-fashioned mold to turn out just before serving.

(Serves 4)
1 package (6-oz.) strawberry-flavored gelatin powder
3 tablespoons Cointreau or your favorite liqueur (optional)
2¼ pounds ripe berries, rinsed, hulled, and sliced

Method: Make the gelatin following the directions on the package, substituting the Cointreau or other liqueur for 3 tablespoons of the water, if you are using. Lay one-third of the prepared berries on the bottom of your glasses or mold. Pour one-third of the gelatin into the glasses or a mold that holds at least 2 pints of liquid and leave to set lightly in the refrigerator. Add another one-third of the berries to the glasses or mold and pour another third of the liquid gelatin on top. Again, leave to set slightly. Repeat a third time, then place in the refrigerator and leave until firmly set.

Serve the dessert in the glasses straight from the refrigerator. To unmold the large dessert, wring out a cloth in boiling water and wrap it around the side and bottom of the mold for a minute, then carefully invert the set gelatin onto a serving plate and give a sharp shake. Lift off the mold.

3. SOW YOUR OATS

Oats have traditionally been used as a tonic to soothe nervous exhaustion, debilitation and depression. Oats? What, that bowl of mushy, beigey, squishy, lumpy mush? Yes, and if you thought that the humble old oat was something you gladly gave up when you left home, think again. This modest food is a force to be reckoned with and you probably have a bag of oats tucked away in the back of your cupboard but have never understood their potential.

Lowers cholesterol

It was 1997 when the US Food and Drug Administration allowed specific health claims to be made about oats in relation to their ability to lower cholesterol. Oats sponge up cholesterol by forming a gel in the small intestine during digestion, and this gel surrounds cholesterol-rich bile acids and prevents them from being reabsorbed into the bloodstream. The trapped bile acids are then eliminated naturally. As a result, the liver pulls more cholesterol out of the bloodstream to make a new supply of bile acids, and blood-cholesterol levels drop. In fact, just one large bowl of oats a day can lower cholesterol according to the FDA.

How this helps fight depression

What does this have to do with depression? Well, by lowering cholesterol you stand a good chance of lowering your risk of depression. There is a link between lower cholesterol and lower cases of depression. High cholesterol levels can cause a narrowing of your arteries which, in turn, leads to poor circulation. This means that the blood that needs to pump around your body is restricted because the cholesterol has deposited fats, which get in the blood's way. The heart has to work harder to get the blood to go round the body and this leaves you feeling depleted of energy and vitality.

But for beating depression, the real winner in oats is the way that this modest grain is able to sustain our blood-sugar levels for longer than any other grain available to us. Oats are able to keep us fuller for longer because they contain complex carbohydrates, which are absorbed into the bloodstream slowly, helping to keep sugar levels stable. Since your body has to work harder to break down the fiber found in complex carbohydrate foods, digestion of the food takes longer. The slowed absorption that results helps provide our bodies with a more stable blood-sugar level and a steady supply of energy. If our sugar levels are stable we are less likely to experience the physical "highs" and "lows" that can make us want to reach for the quick fix of high-sugar/salt/fat food and can make us feel sluggish and depressed. Not only do they sustain us but they are also stimulating and energy-giving. Athletes who have been placed on an oat-based diet show an increase in stamina and oats are now believed to help maintain muscle function during training and exercise.

The nonstop mood booster

Oats not only serve as a great source of fiber but they also provide very useful amounts of protein and iron, which help combat fatigue. They also contain magnesium and zinc, which are brilliant defenses against stress. However, it is the impressive amount of B-vitamins, which help increase the production of the mood booster serotonin, that is the added bonus for anyone suffering from depression. Our levels of serotonin are particularly low in the winter (which can lead to Seasonal Affective Disorder) so making oats a part of your daily routine can be one way of putting a smile on your face.

How to put oats in your diet

✳ Eat a bowl of muesli or porridge for breakfast
✳ Replace breadcrumbs with oats in recipes that need bulk
✳ Eat oat cookies for a snack – easily found in the cookie section of the supermarket
✳ Add oats, instead of flour, to soups to thicken
✳ Replace a third of your flour with oats in recipes requiring plain flour
✳ Buy bread that includes a quantity of oats
✳ Coat chicken or fish with ground oats rather than breadcrumbs
✳ There are recipes for a gorgeous porridge variation called "Oaty Divine" and "Homemade Muesli" in the 7-Day Food Plans under "Breakfast". Here are two more recipes to get those oats working to boost your mood.

APPLE OATY CRUMBLE

(Serves 4)
7 tablespoons walnut or sunflower oil
3 large cooking apples, peeled, cored, and sliced
⅔ cup raisins
1 teaspoon ground cinnamon
6 tablespoons honey
3 cups oatmeal
Greek-style or thick plain yogurt to serve

Method: Heat the oven to 375°F. Place 1 teaspoon of the oil in the bottom of a baking dish suitable for serving from and smear around the bottom and sides. Arrange the apple slices on the bottom of the dish. Sprinkle the raisins and cinnamon on top.

In a saucepan, heat the remaining oil and honey together until the honey melts. Add the oats and mix well. Spoon the oat mixture on top of the apples, spreading it out to cover all the slices. Place the dish in the middle of the oven and bake for 30 minutes. Serve hot with yogurt for spooning over.

MELT-IN-THE-MOUTH OATY PANCAKES

(Makes 12)
⅔ cup wholewheat flour
1 cup rolled oats
1 tablespoon baking powder
1 tablespoon unpasteurized honey
1¼ cups milk
1 egg
2 tablespoons sunflower oil, plus a little extra for cooking
   the pancakes with
1 teaspoon vanilla extract

To serve:
Raw or fresh fruit or fruit preserve
Greek-style or thick plain yogurt

Method: In a large bowl, mix all the dry ingredients together and make a well in the middle. In another bowl, beat the milk and egg together and add the honey and vanilla extract. Pour the milk mixture, a little at a time, into the well in the dry ingredients, beating continuously until the batter just drops off the spoon.

Heat a heavy-bottomed non-stick skillet with a drop of oil over medium-high heat. Drop spoonfuls of the batter onto the skillet and cook the pancakes until small bubbles appear on top and they are golden brown on the bottom. Turn over and continue cooking until golden brown and set. Remove the pancakes from the pan and keep warm in a low oven. Continue making pancakes until all the batter has been used, adding a little extra oil to the pan as necessary. Serve hot with fruit and yogurt.

4. GO NUTS AND FEEL GREAT

We tend to think of nuts as bad for us because we associate them with the things we munch from a dish placed on a bar when we are holding a drink in our other hand. And, yes, those nuts are bad for you – not because they are nuts but because of the way they've been processed. "Roasted, salted peanuts" have unusually high contents of salt and in the case of "honey roasted" nuts, a very high sugar content.

Omega-3 — nutritional inspiration
In their raw state, however, nuts are a natural superfood. All nuts have been found to improve levels of cholesterol because they are an excellent source of omega-3 fatty acids. You can lower your risk of heart disease by up to 25 percent if you eat

a handful of raw, unprocessed nuts five times a week. If you could find a pill that did the same thing, you'd make a fortune. However, a handful of walnuts, for instance, is enough to yield "superfood" benefits. Having a supply of mixed, raw nuts in the kitchen is a great way to snack when you feel the urge to eat between meals. And the omega-3s also offer a benefit for those people who suffer from chronic fatigue, as this useful compound helps strengthen the muscles.

But what's really exciting is the powerful mood-booster effect that omega-3s have. According to research some depression may be caused by omega-3 deficiencies, which result from not eating enough foods that contain the fatty acid, such as nuts. A diet deficient in omega-3s notches up lower levels of the mood-boosting serotonin. Many psychiatrists treat depression with drugs that raise brain levels of serotonin but it also makes sense to boost the body with foods that naturally lift serotonin levels.

Brilliant mood-boosting sustenance

Nuts are brimming with the powerful antioxidant vitamin E called alpha-tocopherol, which is not only excellent for the heart but also helps prevent ageing – this in turn provides the body with more energy to help us fight fatigue. Protein, found in all nuts, is essential for us to build and rebuild organs, muscles, antibodies, hormones and enzymes. Healthy organs, muscles and hormones are particularly important to fight fatigue and exhaustion because if these parts of our bodies are not functioning, this can leave us feeling tired, lethargic and generally depressed. Nuts also contain good levels of zinc, which is a brilliant defense against stress.

Hazelnuts and almonds contain folic acid, which is excellent for supporting the nervous system and helping people who suffer from depression. Brazil nuts are rich in selenium, a trace mineral that is essential to good health but also a terrific mood booster. We only require small amounts of selenium each day, so you really only need to eat three or four Brazil nuts to get the full benefit of this essential mineral. Walnuts are high in folic acid and Vitamin E, both great for lifting the mood. Almonds and cashews contain high levels of iron, which helps fight anemia, an energy-sapping condition. And peanuts are extraordinary protein providers.

When you buy nuts, ensure you always buy whole, raw nuts that have not been salted or processed in any way. You can dry-roast them yourself or leave them in their natural state in a sealed container and dip into them when you need to fill a gap. Leave them on the table for everyone to dip into instead of chips or other high-salt/fat foods. You also can throw them into a blender and chop them up to add to other dishes such as salads and breakfast cereals.

Best nuts for:

depression	stress	chronic fatigue
Brazils	Almonds	Brazils
Peanuts	Pecans	Pecans
Hazel nuts	Brazils	Walnuts
Cashew nuts		

Other ways to go nuts

Peanut butter is a great nut to snack on. Be sure to avoid the mass-market peanut butter as it's full of palm oil, sugar and salt. Instead go to your local health-food shop and get some peanut butter that is pure, without any additives. Spread on a slice of wholewheat bread, rye bread or oat cookies.

Other nut butters, like almond-nut butter, are divine to eat with oat cookies or thrown into a simple stir-fry. Again, you can get these butters from your health-food shop or make your own: take two handfuls of nuts and place them into a blender with a tablespoon of Ace Butter (see page 86) and blend until smooth.

Ground nuts are a sumptuous way to liven up any recipe; simply blend your nuts until they resemble breadcrumbs. Mix into rice or couscous dishes for an added aroma.

Nut creams, such as almond cream, are a gorgeous accompaniment to any sweet dish that would normally require cream — it is delicious with strawberries, for instance.

5. BOOST YOUR MOOD WITH BROCCOLI

Broccoli has received more research than probably any other vegetable because of its powerful cancer-fighting properties. As far as the link between depression and cancer goes, the National Institute of Mental Health (US) states that having cancer can increase your chance of suffering from depression. Interestingly, symptoms of depression can be similar to symptoms of cancer, e.g. a low mood, anxiety, low self-esteem, etc. If you have to take drugs through a cancer treatment, you may also experience some of their powerful side effects, which may also be comparable to depression symptoms, e.g. fatigue, a feeling of hopelessness, unable to concentrate, etc. Broccoli can help fight these symptoms in several ways.

Sulforaphane, the most researched of all broccoli's chemical constituents, helps the body's natural cancer-fighting resources and reduces the risk of developing cancer with its powerful antioxidants and natural detoxifier, according to Johns Hopkins University, a world leader in research and education in medicine and public health based in the US. Hopkins University states that as little as 2 tablespoons of chopped broccoli a day will have a significant effect on helping to combat fatigue, anxiety and stress.

Great for ulcers caused by stress

A common symptom of stress is stomach ulcers. Sulforaphane kills the bacterium known to cause ulcers and when scientists at Johns Hopkins heard that several people had noticed their ulcer symptoms improving after starting to eat broccoli, they investigated. They found that the sulforaphane could succeed where antibiotics failed. Heady words, but the research is proving that, gram for gram, broccoli is perhaps the most powerful ulcer and cancer-fighting superfood and a potent tool in beating chronic stress, anxiety and fatigue, which can lead to stomach problems.

Lightens the load

Broccoli is also high in fiber, which will help the elimination process in the digestive system, and that is vital to our wellbeing because an upset digestive system is a symptom of stress. The nervous system is very sensitive to stress and the state of the nervous system directly affects the digestion process. If you are uptight and anxious you naturally tense your muscles, including those in the digestive region. Added to this, if you are edgy, worried or depressed this can lead to you skipping meals and not taking the time to chew your food; you may eat on the run, grab the first thing that comes to hand or munch on comfort food because you want a quick fix. Both irregular eating and comfort eating can lead to an unhappy digestive system, which in turn can lead to the stress-related diseases that a compacted (constipated) bowel and intestinal tract can bring about, including ulcerative colitis, Crohn's disease and irritable bowel syndrome. So it makes good sense to add two or three portions of this wonderful vegetable to your weekly diet to help your insides cope with your outside world.

Broccoli sprouts for vitality

And if you really want to get the best from broccoli, consider growing some broccoli sprouts. Broccoli sprouts have been found to contain 20–50 times more sulforaphanes than the mature cooked vegetable. This will help you feel more vital, leave you less tired and give you the mood boost you're after. You can grow them in your kitchen (I find they grow easily on the windowsill) and sprinkle them over salad or mix them into any foods so long as you don't cook them.

The ultimate mood booster — folic acid

But for beating the blues, broccoli offers an excellent supply of folic acid. People with depression are more likely to have a folate deficiency and this impairs the metabolism of serotonin — a key player in feeling good. A small handful of raw broccoli offers 100 micrograms of folic acid and the same amount of cooked broccoli offers 50 micrograms of folic acid. Food processing destroys 50—90 percent of the folic acid in foods, as it is very susceptible to heat. If you need a natural lift — quickly — then it is really important to eat the broccoli raw, lightly steamed or stir-fried, as this is the best way to retain its nutrient value. For those people who need a mood boost, an increase of folic acid to 200 micrograms a day will significantly improve your mood and help to lift depression. Folic acid, when introduced to the diet, works best over a long period of time by positively affecting and supporting the nervous system, which helps to counteract stress.

Broccoli also contains:

* More vitamin C than an orange, which boosts the immune system and helps those with chronic fatigue.
* One of the richest sources of vitamin A, which benefits growth, development, reproduction, skin and vision, and will give us an added boost that we so need when we feel out of sorts.
* As much calcium as a glass of milk, which can help relieve mood swings.
* A high amount of flavonoids — which is why broccoli has been singled out as one of the small number of vegetables and fruits that contributes to a significant reduction in heart-disease risk. You are more likely to get heart disease if you are depressed, however you can expect a 20 percent reduction in your risk of heart disease if you eat broccoli.
* More polyphenols — a broad class of antioxidants — than any vegetable except beetroot and red onions. Polyphenol compounds are responsible for the brightly colored pigments of

many fruits and vegetables, as we saw with blueberries, but they also protect plants from diseases and ultraviolet light and the same compounds work in the body to protect against ageing and slowing down, which helps you to fight depression.

✶ Sulfur compounds that help the plant to ward off insects and other mites. If you smell fresh broccoli you will pick up on the slightly sulfurous, bitter smell. Not only does it protect the vegetable but it will also give you a shot of protection every time you eat it.

How to buy and eat

Broccoli is a simple superfood to buy and prepare. It must be picked young to be tender and delicately flavored. Left growing too long, the plant begins converting its sugar to lignin, a type of fiber that continues to be tough even after cooking. If it has been stored too long after harvesting it will be tough and woody. You will know that broccoli is at its best when the florets are green, not purple, and the vegetable is firm, not wilting. Fresh broccoli will have a lovely clean, green smell.

To get the best from broccoli, eat it raw by dipping it into some houmous, red pepper dip, tzatziki (see recipe below) or your favorite dip. An effortless way to cook broccoli is to steam it, dribble over some vinaigrette or a knob of butter and serve it as an accompaniment to a meal.

BROCCOLI WITH A TZATZIKI DIP

Serve this traditional Greek mouthwatering dip with raw broccoli flowerets, cauliflower flowerets, carrot slices, and celery sticks.

(Makes about 1½cups)
1 cup Greek-style or thick plain yogurt
½ cucumber, seeded and coarsely grated

Grated peel and juice of 1 lemon
1 clove of garlic, crushed

A pinch of cayenne pepper

Method: Mix all ingredients together, adjusting the cayenne to taste. Cover and chill until required.

BROCCOLI DRIZZLED WITH HONEY, CHILI AND SESAME SAUCE

Lightly cooked, tender broccoli is delicious drizzled with this sweet dressing – it really soaks into the flowerets so each mouthful is well flavored and juicy.

(Serves 4)
12 ounces fresh broccoli, trimmed
2 tablespoons olive oil
1 tablespoon honey
1 teaspoon light soy sauce
1 small fresh red chili, seeded and chopped
1 tablespoon sesame seeds, toasted, to garnish

Method: Bring a pan of water to a boil. Add the broccoli and continue boiling for 5 minutes, or until you can easily slide a sharp knife into a stem.

Meanwhile, in a small bowl, mix together all the other ingredients, except the sesame seeds. Drain the broccoli and place it on a serving platter. Drizzle the dressing over while the broccoli is still warm, and finish with a sprinkling of sesame seeds.

BROCCOLI PENNE WITH CASHEW NUTS

This is a perfect supper dish you can throw together in minutes. It helps you out of a tricky moment when you get home and everyone is hungry. Buy a good-quality penne pasta; it only costs a few cents more but tastes so much nicer than cheaper brands.

(Serves 4)
1 pound dried penne or other tube shapes
1 pound broccoli
4 tablespoons olive oil
1 clove of garlic, crushed
Juice of 1 lemon
4 ounces toasted cashew nuts

Method: Bring a large saucepan of water to a boil, then add the pasta and boil for 10 minutes, or according to the cooking directions on the package, until the pasta is just tender to the bite. At the same time, place the broccoli in a steamer over another pan of boiling water and steam for about 10 minutes, or until the broccoli is very tender.

Meanwhile, gently heat the oil in a saucepan or skillet large enough to hold all the ingredients and add the garlic to soften. When the broccoli is tender, drain it well and break it up with a fork or mash it with a potato masher. Add the broccoli to the pan with the garlic over low heat. Drain the pasta and gently stir it into the pan with the broccoli. Add the lemon juice and stir for about one minute to let the flavors infuse. Finally, stir in the cashews and serve.

6. THE HOT TOMATO

There are few fruits which have commanded so much media attention focusing on their health benefits in the last few years. The research that has come out about the tomato is exciting and inspiring and nothing has been hotter than the studies about its lycopene. Lycopene is a carotenoid, a chemical compound that is found in fruit and vegetables and gives the yellow, orange or red color to them. The lycopene found in tomatoes (and everything made from them) has been extensively studied for its antioxidant and cancer-preventing properties. The antioxidant function of lycopene has been linked to the prevention of heart disease, some types of cancer and boosting the immune system. Because depression and stress can give our immune system a huge dent, sometimes resulting in chronic fatigue, it's important that we eat powerful foods to build our strength up, because the age-old symptoms that arise as a result of a lack of antioxidants do include tiredness, depression and feeling old.

The lycopene that has been the subject of such hot gossip is found predominately in the skin of the tomato and is what gives the tomato its rich red color. This compound protects the skin of the tomato from the harsh rays of the sun and, when you think about it, you can see how it works. Even though tomatoes sit in the sun for days, sometimes weeks, their skin still stays wrinkle-free and undamaged, and this is thought to be due to the antioxidants in the lycopene. Furthermore, the bigger the ratio of skin to flesh, the more lycopene there is in the tomato; so cherry tomatoes, gram for gram, have more lycopene than big tomatoes. Because the job of the lycopene is to protect the tomato's skin from the sun's harsh rays, so it is thought that this sun defense in the tomato is also brilliant for strengthening our own skins' sun defenses. This powerful defense can help protect our cells both outside and inside the body. Protecting our cells helps to slow down the ageing system and this will help us feel less like "old bones" and help build our bodies up — essential in fighting depression. Eating energy-building foods like tomatoes rather than energy-depleting foods like sugar can help strengthen us and encourage us to feel better.

The canned ones are even better
What's even more exciting about tomatoes is that cooked tomatoes release five times more lycopene than raw ones. This is because tomatoes are mostly water, so when cooked the lycopene becomes more concentrated; added to that this magic substance is also more easily absorbed into the system when it is cooked. And, yes, we are talking about the canned variety; it

isn't often we can state that canned vegetables or fruit are better for you than fresh ones. The thrust behind cooked tomatoes as a superfood is the amount of lycopene in them per gram; there are 27mg in 2 tablespoons of tomato purée, but about half that in a large slice of watermelon, which is the nearest rival for lycopene content. We should take in 22mg of lycopene a day for its optimal benefits. If, like me, you can give the hard, under-ripe tomatoes in the shops a miss, this offers a different way to view tomatoes and ways that we can eat them.

The folate mood boost

Another ingredient of the tomato which may help those suffering from depression is the vitamin folate. Research carried out on folate at the US Tufts University in 2003 showed that those who suffered from major depression had lower concentrations of folate in their bloodstream, and particularly their red blood cells, than those who had never been depressed. A lack of folate is said to cause irritability, mental fatigue, insomnia, muscular fatigue as well as depression. Because a lack of folate is linked to a lack of red blood cells, it seems appropriate that the rich, red tomato might be able to infuse our bodies with some of this productive vitamin and help us to regain our strength and fortitude.

Stress-busting vitamin C

Vitamin C is also present in tomatoes and this is important particularly if you suffer from stress. Stress can deplete the body of vitamin C, which can then produce depression. This is described as vitamin C anemia and causes the body to absorb less iron, which in turn renders the body tired and worn out. A lack of vitamin C can also result in muscle weakness, a common symptom of chronic fatigue. It is therefore a good boost to the system and, together with their lycopene and folate, cooked tomatoes eaten three times a week can be a powerful tool in fighting depression and its ongoing symptoms.

The classic tomato sauce is a good way to get started in integrating some of the formidable tomato talents into our daily food plan for beating depression, fatigue and stress.

THE SIMPLEST AND BEST TOMATO SAUCE

No need to mess with this recipe; it really is as simple as it looks.

(Serves 4)
2 cans (15-oz,) crushed tomatoes
6 tablespoons olive oil
Handful of fresh basil leaves

Method: Place the tomatoes with their juices into a pan over low heat and simmer for 15 minutes, stirring occasionally, or until thick and glossy. Stir in the olive oil and continue heating for 5 minutes longer.

Meanwhile, chop the basil leaves finely and add to the tomato mixture just before taking the sauce off the heat. To serve, pour the sauce over freshly cooked pasta, freshly steamed vegetables or rice; spoon it over a pizza base and add sliced onions, bell peppers, and mushrooms for a really healthy pizza; pour it over fresh fish and oven bake; or mix with cooked, lean ground beef and fried chopped onions to make a delicious ragú sauce.

MEDITERRANEAN TOMATO TART

This is one of the most tempting ways I know to turn cherry tomatoes into a mood-boosting party piece of a meal.

(Serves 4)
1 can (15-oz.) crushed tomatoes
5 cups sliced onions
4 tablespoons olive oil
½ pound cherry or baby plum tomatoes

12 ounces puff pastry dough, thawed if frozen
½ cup pitted green olives, chopped
3 cloves of garlic, crushed
2 teaspoons fresh oregano, chopped, or 1 teaspoon dried
⅓ cup freshly grated Pecorino Romano cheese, plus extra for sprinkling over at the table
Tossed green salad to serve

Method: Heat the oven to 400°F. Put the canned tomatoes and their juices into a heavy-bottomed saucepan over medium heat and simmer until reduced by one-third. Meanwhile, in a large skillet, fry the onions in the olive oil until they are soft and see-through. Place the cherry/baby plum tomatoes on top and cover and cook on a medium heat until their skins have broken and they are soft.

Roll out the puff pastry dough on a lightly floured surface and place onto a lightly greased 16- x 12-inch baking tray. Add the olives, garlic and oregano to the tomato sauce and mix well. Spoon this over the dough. Arrange the onions and baby tomatoes on top.

Place in the oven and bake for about 20 minutes. Remove from the oven and sprinkle the top with the cheese, then place back into the oven for 5 minutes longer. Cut into slices and serve hot or lukewarm with extra cheese for sprinkling over and a salad on the side.

ROAST TOMATO RISOTTO

A stunning risotto and a powerful mood meal.

(Serves 4)
1 pound tomatoes
6 tablespoons olive oil
1 small butternut squash
1 onion, finely chopped
Scant 1½ cups good-quality risotto rice

1¼ cups chicken or vegetable stock
1¼ cups dry white wine
1 bunch of fresh flat-leaf parsley, chopped
Pinch of dried sage
3 cloves of garlic, crushed
⅓ cup freshly grated Pecorino Romano cheese

Method: Heat the oven to 400°F. Place the tomatoes on a baking tray and drizzle them with 3 tablespoons of the olive oil. Roast the tomatoes for 30 minutes until they are well cooked, soft, and squishy. Meanwhile, peel the squash and chop the flesh into small pieces.

Place the remaining olive oil in a large, heavy-bottomed saucepan and gently fry the squash and onion until they are soft. Add the tomatoes and mix, then stir in the rice and garlic and stir the whole mixture for 2 minutes. Add enough stock to just cover the rice and continue stirring while the rice absorbs the stock, about 5 minutes. Add more stock to just cover the rice and continue stirring until it is absorbed. When all the stock has been used, continue adding wine, little by little, until all the liquid is absorbed.

Now, stir in the herbs, and cheese and continue to stir over low heat for 2 minutes. Serve immediately – this dish needs no accompaniment!

7. PARSLEY POWER

Parsley is one of those herbs you hardly notice yet it contains some potent and nutrimental goodness which will help in combating depression and fighting stress.

A vibrant tonic
First and foremost, parsley is a nurturing, warming, vibrant mood-boosting tonic. It is a well-known fact that if you like roses you

should plant parsley alongside them to encourage good health and a gorgeous fragrance from your blooms. Likewise, if you are suffering from depression, stress or fatigue, adding this illustrious herb to your diet could act as a tonic for your mood.

Parsley has traditionally been used as a digestive-tract tonic, for bladder infections, as a blood cleanser and a boost for the liver and kidneys. It has also, unconventionally, been used as a remedy to help animals after giving birth by helping a mother dog or cat stop lactating. It aids with afterbirth pains and can generally help get them back on their feet. But for people who suffer from depression, eating parsley can bring about the benefits from the abundant supply of the dynamic B-vitamins.

Vitamin B

For a powerful mood-strengthening tonic, it's the high concentration of B-vitamins that make parsley so dynamic for beating depression, fatigue and stress. Generally speaking, vitamin B consists of a combination of vitamins that comprise what is known as the B-complex vitamins. Deficiencies in the B-vitamins can lead to memory loss, fatigue, irritability, anxiety, mental slowness and mental confusion. These vitamins work most effectively when combined – each playing a central role. As parsley has a high count of the B-vitamins, incorporating this herb into your diet can help to act as a tonic to your mental fitness. Here is a quick overview of these great vitamins.

* B1, or thiamine, enhances circulation, thought activity and brain function. Deficiencies in this vitamin can result in fatigue, weak muscles, nerve damage and stress.
* B2, or riboflavin, helps the body release energy from foods, which helps to combat the symptoms of chronic fatigue.
* B3, or niacin, contributes to the proper functioning of the central nervous system, which helps strengthen us – vital for when we are stressed.
* B6, or pyridoxine, aids in the metabolism and absorption of

protein and assists in red blood cell formation, both of which help to increase your energy. B6 is also important in the synthesis of neurotransmitters, the chemicals that transmit information from and within the brain, which are essential to feeling good.

✳ B12 is necessary for energy production and the maintenance of the nervous system, which is paramount for fighting depression. There is more evidence linking a deficiency of B12 to depression than any other B-vitamin, which is why it's so important for us to get a good supply of this vital vitamin.

Phytoestrogens to ease the monthly blues

The second exquisiteness of parsley is that it is Mother Nature's helping hand for women's menstrual cycle. It has been said that parsley helps to ease the menstrual cycle by soothing premenstrual tension and nerves, acting as a natural diuretic for bloating, stimulating the uterus and relieving headaches and cramps. As a natural blood tonic, parsley also helps by stimulating and regulating delayed, clotted or irregular blood flow. This is due to the phytoestrogens that are found in parsley. These are compounds found in plants that produce an oestrogen-like effect in the body but come as a safe and natural compound. When oestrogen levels are higher in the body, this can help to combat the tiredness and fatigue that comes with the menstrual cycle.

Vitamin C, the super vitamin for depression

Parsley also contains vitamin C, more than any other vegetable or fruit, ounce for ounce. Vitamin C is a super vitamin for fighting depression. Because it acts as an antioxidant and helps to maintain the immune system, manufacture collagen, guard against cancer and heart disease, its presence in the body encourages good health and vitality. Equally, a lack of vitamin C can lead to depression and mental confusion, amongst other problems.

Glutamine – helps get the goodness to the brain

Glutamine is an amino acid that can help lift depression. Parsley contains glutamine, but it is easily destroyed by cooking, so the best recipes to ensure the highest amount of glutamine use parsley in its raw state.

Although flat-leaved parsley has become popular in our modern recipes, it is actually the thick, dark, curly-headed parsley which is the majestic superfood. This variety of parsley is much richer and denser in nutrients. When you buy a bunch of parsley, place it in a vase filled with water, just as you would do with a bunch of flowers. The parsley will keep fresher for longer than if you simply place it in the refrigerator.

PARSLEY AND ALMOND PATÉ

A delicious mix of fresh parsley and mood-boosting almonds. Simply spread it on your favorite wholewheat toast.

1 red bell pepper, cored, seeded, and thickly sliced
1⅓ cups blanched almonds
1 large bunch of fresh curly parsley, rinsed and stems removed
1⅓ cups green olives, pitted
Juice of 1 lemon
7 tablespoon olive oil
Wholewheat toast to serve

Method: Heat the broiler to high. Place the pepper under the broiler and broil until soft. Toast the almonds in a dry skillet until the color just slightly darkens – but don't let them burn. Wash the parsley and remove the stalks. Place all the ingredients in a blender and blend until smooth.

PARSLEY PESTO

This rich parsley sauce also incorporates walnuts, which will give you the added benefits of "brain-boosting" omega-3s.

⅔ cup shelled walnuts
1 large bunch of curly parsley, rinsed and largest stems
  removed
2 cloves of garlic, peeled
7 tablespoons walnut oil or olive oil
Finely grated peel and juice of 1 lemon

Method: Toast the walnuts in a dry skillet over medium-high heat until just brown; immediately tip the walnuts into a blender. Add the remaining ingredients to the blender and blend until smooth. To serve, add a large portion of the pesto to some freshly cooked wholewheat pasta or *just-steamed* rice.

8. GIVE A FIG

There are some good reasons why these dazzling fruits are a superfood for helping to fight fatigue, depression and stress. But best of all — they're so delicious! But the two areas that concern those of us who are eating for better mental health are potassium and fiber.

Potassium — a vital mineral to boost alertness and build up strength

Figs are high in potassium, which is a mineral essential for the proper functioning of cell growth, nervous-system tissue and for muscle building. In the body it is classified as an electrolyte (meaning it turns into ions, which is good for cells) and performs various functions including protein synthesis (when a cell gets a message to make protein) and regulation of fluids in body tissue. The reason we need a good supply of potassium is that stress depletes it from our bodies and, according to the British Medical Association (BMA), this can create muscle weakness, which can lead to chronic fatigue and impairs our concentration. Muscle weakness is commonly associated with chronic fatigue and that achy, tired feeling can really pull your mood down. The BMA also states that a lack of potassium can also lead to poor concentration and this can leave you feeling fuzzy and disorientated, which is associated with depression and stress. So eating a couple of figs a day could help to stop the cycle of stress/depression/fatigue that comes with a potassium deficiency.

Fiber – essential for beating that sluggish feeling

Figs are also high in dietary fiber. A study at Cardiff University, Wales, in 2002 revealed that a diet that includes a higher amount of fibre than the average diet has a marked effect on our mental wellbeing. After just one week of the trial starting, the results were astonishing as the subjects showed a 10 percent reduction in fatigue, lower depression scores and better cognitive powers — the way we think and learn. The study by Professor Andrew Smith revealed that people who ate a diet high in fiber were also less stressed.

These findings make sense because if we don't eat enough fiber, our digestive systems struggle to eliminate waste food. Once our systems are struggling, our bodies use a lot more energy as they have to work so much harder, and this makes us tired. Not only that but there is a fantastic feeling that goes with a high intake of good fiber because you feel cleaner inside, which helps you to feel lighter and more mentally buoyant. It is recommended by the US Food and Drugs Administration that we eat 25g of fiber a day, yet our average intake is nearer 12g a day. One fresh fig will give you 2g of natural, wholesome, nutritious fiber, which can go a long way to helping you feel more vibrant, less stressed and more bright and breezy.

Get into dried figs, too

Figs have a short shelf life — about a week — which is why so many are dried. Generally speaking, buy dried figs which are plump and not too dried out. Dried figs are very high in natural sugars and are the perfect antidote to beat those sugar cravings; reaching for three figs instead of a chocolate bar can help avoid the "sugar crash" that comes about half an hour after eating chocolate or another high-sugar food and will help level out mood swings. For a fruit, figs are also exceptionally high in iron, and getting as much iron from your food as you can is important to keep anemia at bay, especially if you suffer from tiredness or chronic fatigue. For fiber, five dried figs will give you 50 percent of the recommended daily intake of fiber — now that's worth giving a fig for!

FRESH FIGS WITH ORANGE SYRUP

The fig season is very short, so don't let it pass you by. Here is a gorgeous recipe for making the most of this luxurious fruit.

(Serves 4)
1¼ cups freshly squeezed orange juice
2-inch piece of fresh ginger root, grated without peeling first
2 star anise
12 fresh figs

Method: Put the orange juice, ginger, and star anise in a saucepan and bring to a boil. Reduce the heat and simmer for 30 minutes, stirring occasionally, or until a light syrup forms. Strain the syrup and discard the remains.

Slice the figs in half and arrange on serving plates. Drizzle the orange syrup over the figs and serve hot or chilled.

FIGGIE FLAPJACKS

These delicious flapjacks are both yummy and healthy, as well as a virtuous sweet snack or dessert.

(Makes 8)
7 tablespoons sunflower oil
7 tablespoons (scant 1 stick) butter

3 tablespoons unpasteurized honey
3¾ cups rolled oats
7 ounces dried figs, chopped into small pieces with the
  middle stems discarded
3½ tablespoons orange juice
2 tablespoons brandy (optional)

Method: Heat the oven to 350ºF. Dribble a little of the sunflower oil in a 5-inch square baking pan; set aside. Melt the butter with the remaining oil in a heavy-bottomed saucepan. Stir in the honey and when it melts thoroughly stir in the rolled oats. Spoon half the mixture into the baking pan and spread out to cover the bottom of the pan. Place in the oven and bake for 10 minutes, or until the top turns a golden brown. Meanwhile, place the figs in a pan with the orange juice and brandy and simmer gently until the figs are soft and the liquid is syrupy. When the tray of oat mixture is golden brown, spoon the figgy mixture over and then top with the remaining oat mixture so you have a "sandwich" effect.

Return the pan to the oven and bake for 15 minutes longer, or until the oats on the top are golden brown. Remove the pan from the oven and set on a wire rack to cook. Cut into squares to serve. Everyone will love this delicious treat!

9. THE NURTURING AVOCADO

How can anything so delicious also be such a good-for-you food? Avocados are full of mood-boosting nutrition which can help beat depression and simultaneously nurture the palate. That soft, subtle and creamy flesh offers so much more than a salad extra!

Good-for-you fats

Let's first look at the fatty issue. Avocados are naturally rich in omega-3 and a diet rich in this magic fat is wholly beneficial to the body if we suffer from depression. The evidence is palpable that it will boost your mood. Harvard researcher Andrew Stoll found doses of omega-3 fatty acids improved symptoms of manic depression in 64 percent of 14 patients after 4 months against 18 percent of those on a placebo. Stoll conjectures that omega-3 fat affects signalling among brain cells in much the same way that drugs for treating manic depression do.

The calorie issue

Before you say "but they're so fattening," let's look at the calorie issue; because whilst we are loving the avocado, there is the concern about the amount of calories that it contains, so our modern infatuation with losing weight may have put us off eating this nourishing fruit. Below is a list that gives an indication of the amount of calories in an avocado in comparison to other foods:

Food	Calories per 100g
White Bread Roll	280
Special K	369
Ready Salted Chips	470
Banana	95
Avocado	190

The avocado is high in calories compared with other fruit, which don't contain omega-3 fats, but compared with other everyday foods it is very low in calories. Avocados are brilliant at satisfying that craving for creamy, high-fat foods that we are so fond of and find so hard to resist. So whilst you are on the 7-Day Food Plan, eat an avocado a day as part of your "five a day" fruit and vegetables to help you beat those cravings and stay on the straight and narrow.

Nutrient booster – great for absorbing additional nutrients

A second bonus for the fats found in the avocado was discovered and published in the *Journal of Nutrition*, March 2005, and indicated that the fats found specifically in avocados act as a "nutrient booster" and increase the body's ability to absorb and use carotenoids. Carotenoids are powerful antioxidants that help protect the body from damaging compounds. They also allow the body to absorb significantly more heart-healthy nutrients like alphacarotene, betacarotene and lycopene, which are generally found in fruits and vegetables. Because many fruits and vegetables rich in carotenoids are also fat-free, this may limit the body's ability to absorb some of these nutrients and specifically antioxidants.

When we are depressed or suffer from chronic fatigue, what we need is a good supply of antioxidants to build up our strength and help us resist the stress that comes with feeling low. Avocados help the body build itself up whilst offering up the most delicious natural food at the same time.

Lecithin – helping us break down fats

Avocados are also an excellent source of the wonderful compound, lecithin, which is a type of fatty acid. This superb fatty substance is used by the body to help break down fats in the diet, and also helps form substances vital for transmission of nerve impulses and the creation of healthy nervous tissue. It is needed by every cell in the body and is a key building block of cell membranes; without it, they would harden. Lecithin protects cells from oxidation and largely makes up the protective sheaths surrounding the brain. This wonderful fatty matter is also a boost to the brain and, in turn, helps to reduce anxiety and depression.

Just take them naked

A ripe avocado eaten scooped out of its skin with a spoon is such a lovely but simple snack. Have a bowl of avocados on your kitchen table. As they take three to four days to ripen, it's best to buy them in advance because when the recipe calls for an avocado, you don't want to pay over the odds for the "sun ripened" ones in the shops when you can do just as well at home. Here are two sumptuous recipes to create that are good enough for the most sophisticated palate and offer you a mood boost in one fell swoop.

AVOCADO SALSA

This spicy, tangy dip can be served with vegetable crudités to give you a piquant snack or as a first course. It helps your body devour the good nutrients from all the other ingredients.

(Serves 4)
3 ripe tomatoes
6 scallions, finely chopped
2 ripe avocados, peeled, stoned, and finely chopped
1 small bunch cilantro, stems removed and leaves finely chopped
1 green chili, seeded and sliced
Freshly squeezed juice of 1 lime
A good selection of prepared raw vegetables to serve

Method: Stick the tomatoes, one at a time, onto the end of a fork and place into a pan of boiling water for 1 minute. Once they have cooled to the touch, peel their skins off, scrape out the seeds, and chop the flesh into small pieces. Mix all the ingredients together, then cover and leave them to marinate in the refrigerator for an hour or so before serving. Serve with peeled and sliced vegetables.

AVOCADOS WITH WHOLEWHEAT PENNE

A great meal you can't beat for its high nutrition content and its delicious energy-giving nourishment.

(Serves 4)

1 pound dried penne or other tube shapes

6 tablespoons olive oil

1 large onion, finely chopped

1 red bell pepper, cored, seeded, and sliced

2 cloves of garlic, crushed

1½ cups drained and chopped sun-dried tomatoes in oil

1 small bunch of fresh cilantro

2 avocados, peeled, stoned and chopped

Pecorino Romano or feta cheese to serve

Method: Bring a large pan of water to a boil. Add the pasta and boil for 10 minutes, or according to the directions on the package, until tender to the bite.

Meanwhile, place 4 tablespoons of the olive oil in a heavy-bottomed saucepan and heat gently. Add the onion and leave it to sweat until it is transparent. Add the pepper and continue cooking for 3 minutes, stirring occasionally, or until the pepper is just soft. Add the garlic and cook for one minute longer. When the pasta is tender, drain it well and immediately place in a large serving dish. Pour over the onion, pepper, and garlic mixture. Add all the other ingredients and gently toss together. Serve with freshly grated Pecorino Romano cheese or crumbled feta cheese for sprinkling over the top.

10. HONEY – THE BEE'S KNEES

Honey is one of nature's gifts and, for fighting depression, there can be no food that is more nurturing than rich and fabulous honey. Honey is the perfect food to eat when you are craving sugar and, as you will see further down, it carries none of the dispiriting effects that eating sugar will give you.

Energy booster

Honey is one of nature's loving foods and the phrase "as sweet as honey" sums up how we feel about honey as an adorable and benevolent food that does not strip us of anything. Honey is absorbed straight into the bloodstream without needing to be digested. The nutrients from honey can be found in the blood as quickly as two hours after being eaten. When we eat honey we can feel more energy, but, unlike sugar, it doesn't give us that "sugar low" because it doesn't affect the body's glucose levels in the same way. Athletes often eat honey before training to give them extra energy and, if you feel tired and worn down, this could help to give you the lift you are looking for.

Immune booster

Honey also contains small amounts of antioxidants, which are powerful phytochemicals to help boost your immune system. According to research presented at the American Chemical Society in Anaheim, California, in March 2004, daily consumption of honey raises blood levels of protective antioxidants — a direct link was found between the research subjects' honey consumption and the level of antioxidants in their blood. When we are run down and depressed or stressed we want as many antioxidants as we can to help us get our energy and strength back up to full quota.

Manuka honey

However, there is honey and there is manuka honey. Manuka honey is made by bees which gather pollen from the flowers of the manuka bush, which is indigenous to New Zealand. The honey-making process is enriched by the pollution-free environment of New Zealand, and certain types of manuka honey have been observed to have some very special properties indeed. Manuka honey is the only honey that has been tested for its antibacterial activity and it has been found that it has a terrific antimicrobial agent which kills or inhibits the growth of micro-organisms but causes little or no host damage. We want plenty of these in our diets because when we are depressed we are more likely to pick up viruses and bacterial infections, so including a good source of antimicrobial agents will strengthen our backup systems. The antimicrobial agent also inhibits against bacteria, which can cause stomach ulcers, a prevalent symptom of modern-day stress.

Manuka honey can be found in health-food shops and it is given a number according to how "active" it is in antimicrobial agents. The higher the number, the more active; buy what you can afford and bear in mind what it is replacing, for instance, in my case, several bars of chocolate and expensive ice cream!

Beat the sugar cravings

What I have found with honey is that a teaspoonful of this gorgeous nectar will kill off any sugar cravings that I experience in moments of stress. I know that if I go for the chocolate bar I will regret it an hour later but, in all these situations, it pays to be prepared. I always keep a jar of cold-pressed, local honey and if the need arises, I have my elixir for nipping a "sugar roll" on the head. It only takes a teaspoonful on an oat cookie to hit the spot and that's what makes it such a powerful superfood to help fight depression with food.

Here are a couple of recipes that will also give you the sweetness of the honey and a delicious mood boost as well.

SOOTHY SMOOTHIE

This nutritious smoothie is good for breakfast or a pick-me-up after work. Just give it a try and feel the honey energize you and the banana soothe you.

(Makes 2 smoothies)
1 mango or papaya, peeled, seeded, and chopped
1 medium banana, peeled
1 tablespoon tahini (sesame-seed paste)
½ cup fruit juice
1tbsp/15ml honey
⅔ cup plain yogurt with live bacteria

Method: Put all the ingredients into a blender and blend until smooth. This will sort you out! (Remember to discard the seeds of the papaya; I put them in a smoothie once and felt sick all day!)

FIG AND APRICOT COMPOTE

This luscious compote will satisfy everyone's sweet tooth, while offering the benefits of the dried fruit — lots of minerals and fiber!

(Serves 4)
Juice of 1 lemon
Juice of 2 oranges
⅔ cup sliced dried apricots
⅔ cup chopped dried figs
⅓ cup raisins
2 tablespoons unpasteurized honey
Fresh fruit to serve
½ cup chopped toasted walnuts

Method: Place the lemon and orange juices in a saucepan and bring to a boil. Add the apricots, figs, and raisins, reduce heat to low, and simmer for about 10 minutes until they become tender, but still whole, and the juices are a little syrupy. Use a slotted spoon to remove the fruit and reduce the sauce until it is even thicker, about 5 minutes longer.

Remove the pan from the heat and leave the syrup to cool a little. Return the apricots, figs, and raisins to the sauce, then add the walnuts and honey. Serve warm or chilled spooned over fresh fruit.

6
THE 7-DAY
FOOD
PLANS

FINDING THE RIGHT PLAN FOR YOU

Here are three questionnaires for depression, stress and chronic fatigue to help you to decipher which food plan is best for you. Score one point for each "yes" and the questionnaire which reveals the most points is probably the right Food Plan for you to follow.

Are you depressed?

✻ Do you have a low mood and feel sad or cry a lot?
✻ Have you lost interest in activities and other people you once enjoyed?
✻ Have you experienced changes in sleeping pattern?
✻ Do you feel tired, or even exhausted, when you wake up?
✻ Do you have feelings of guilt or feel ashamed?
✻ Do you regularly feel nervous, anxious and agitated?
✻ Are you unable to concentrate or remember things?
✻ Have other people noticed a change in you?
✻ Do you feel hopeless, or worthless?
✻ Are you easily overwhelmed by stress or worry?
✻ Have you experienced changes in weight?
✻ Are you exceptionally critical of yourself and others?
✻ Do you find it difficult to make decisions?
✻ Have you lost interest in eating good food?
✻ Do you feel hostile toward others?
✻ Are you keeping a secret that you feel you can't let out?

Are you stressed?

✻ Do you feel that you cannot achieve your goals?
✻ Do you feel physically run down?
✻ Are you angry at others for making demands?
✻ Do you berate yourself for putting up with those demands?
✻ Do you feel an increase in muscle tension?
✻ Are you more sarcastic or negative than usual?
✻ Do you blow up over minor issues?

* Is your digestion a problem? (E.g. more stomach aches, indigestion, etc.)
* Do you feel overwhelmed at the moment?
* Are you having trouble sleeping well?
* Has your blood pressure increased?
* Are you experiencing more headaches than usual?
* Has your sex drive decreased?
* Are you feeling lonely?
* Are you taking more risks than normal?
* Are you overly suspicious or jealous?

Are you chronically fatigued?
* Do you feel tired most of the time?
* Do your muscles ache?
* Does your fatigue interfere with your daily activities?
* Are your glands sore?
* Do you become exhausted after a small task?
* Do you struggle to focus on your tasks?
* Are you beginning to think that your chronic fatigue is never going to go?
* Do you feel tired after a night's sleep?
* Do you have problem remembering things?
* Do you pick up colds easily?
* Do you feel like sleeping in the afternoon?
* Do you get more headaches than you used to?
* Do your joints hurt?
* Do you feel angry with yourself for being so tired?
* Can you not be bothered to get angry or feel full of joy?
* Do you sometimes feel a little better, try to do something that used to be easy and find yourself more exhausted?

If you find that the scores for each of these questionnaires are similar and you don't know which plan to begin, the Depression Food Plan is a good plan to start with as it will give you more energy and boost your mood, both of which will ease stress.

GETTING STARTED

This section takes you through three separate food plans that have been designed to help beat depression, fatigue or stress, and there are some general guidelines that apply to all three plans.

PREPARATION

The key to maintaining any good food plan is in the preparation. The key preparation points are as follows:

Shopping
* Ensure you have the foods you need in your house at least the day before you plan to eat them. The exception to this is if you have to soak any pulses overnight and then you need to have these in two days before you eat in order to have enough soaking and cooking time.
* It is easier to purchase all your dried foods for the week at once and then you only need to shop for your meat/fish and vegetables on the day before you eat them.
* The more prepared you are the less likely you are to pop into the shops and become seduced by something else that looks tasty but is not included in the food plan.

Cooking
The food plans are designed so that you can prepare your lunch the night before. This means that minimal effort is required on the day if you are dashing out of the door first thing.

Transportation
The lunches are designed to be transportable for those people who need to take a meal with them. Investment in a wide-mouthed flask is a good idea if you eat at work because a hot, home-cooked meal is satisfying and nurturing, and this in itself will help you to sail through your afternoon.

Calories

If you are a calorie counter, you don't need to count calories this week. If you are overweight, what's more important is that you get into a food rhythm and routine and enjoy cooking for your emotional wellbeing rather than measuring your food intake. If you find that at the end of the week you are feeling better then you may be more inclined to nurture your way through weight loss with a balanced eating regime rather than forcing yourself to endure a punishing schedule. Let your hunger be your guide. My grandmother used to say, "Leave the table wanting one more mouthful."

Madcap moment

We all have a time in the day when we need a "food prop" time to keep us going. For Joan it's the 3.30 p.m. "just got back from picking the kids up from school and flagging" and for Ian it's the 6.30 p.m. "home from work and need something straight away" moment. In all cases you can have good food ready for these occasions, such as a bowl of home-made fruit salad or a bag of prepared crudités in the fridge. It is very important to have food ready for these moments because these are our "madcap moments" when nothing is going to stand between us and our snack – but we are more likely to dive into a great snack if it's ready, otherwise we end up diving into a bag of chips or something worse!

Snacks

Here are some snacks that will satisfy you in a madcap moment:

✱ Fruit salad — always have one prepared in the refrigerator (see the recipe under Breakfast).
✱ A handful of mixed nuts — a mixture of unsalted nuts help overcome the craving for high-calorie foods. Almonds, cashews, brazil and walnuts all contain:

- Folic acid – helps alleviate depression
- Zinc – boosts immune system
- Magnesium – to fight stress
- Selenium – to boost your mood

✽ A handful of seeds. My favourite mixture is as follows: take 1 cup each of sunflower, pumpkin, sesame seeds and pine nuts, and place them all in a heavy-bottomed pan. Place on the heat and dry-toast the seeds without burning. When cooled put into a sealed container and take a handful when necessary. This mixture will last you the week.

✽ A cupful of muesli – without milk.

✽ A piece of fruit – remember to top yourself up to at least five portions of fruit and vegetables a day. Here is a quick look at what fruit is good for what:
  - Banana – stress-busting qualities
  - Kiwi – boost of vitamin C – good for fighting fatigue
  - Apples – great for a sluggish digestion and lowering cholesterol
  - Pear – contains copper and is a good fruit for beating the sugar craving
  - Mandarin/tangerine – good for fighting irritability
  - Berries – simply star boosters – eat a handful a day
  - Melon – contains stress-busting magnesium and is great for beating a sugar craving

✽ Unsalted oat cookies (can be easily purchased from any supermarket).

✽ Crudités – always have a bag of prepared raw carrots, celery, peppers or your favorite vegetables; a handful constitutes one portion of your daily five.

✽ Unsalted rice cakes.

✽ Dried fruit – figs, apricots and dates are especially delicious.

Flexibility

The meals have been planned with a busy lifestyle in mind. The lunches are meant to be simple with the suppers being more lavish. However, if your lifestyle dictates that you eat a leisurely lunch and a simple supper, just turn the meals around the other way. Conversely, if you would prefer to swap one day's meals with another, feel free to be flexible; just ensure that you eat all the meals included in the food plan.

Freezing

Mostly, the meals are for four portions unless otherwise stated. Don't hesitate to make extra and freeze the meals ready for a stressful moment when you cannot manage to cook. It feels so good to open the freezer, knowing that there's a home-cooked meal only a "defrost" moment away.

Fish

There are several fish recipes in the food plans; if you don't like the fish in that recipe or that particular fish is unavailable, change it for fish that is available or which you would prefer to eat.

Your choices are: salmon, tuna, mackerel, herring, sardines, pilchards, swordfish and orange roughy. Eat the fish whole or filleted – the choice is yours.

BREAKFAST FOR ALL

Breakfast is the most important meal there is. In order to have your sugar levels balanced you need to eat some nourishing food early on, and this will help you get the power boost you need to start the day. Here is a selection of breakfasts from which you can choose the ones that appeal to your taste buds the most. It doesn't matter which food plan you are following – just choose your breakfasts from the following selection.

FRESH FRUIT SALAD

Fresh fruits are high energy foods that offer get-up-and-go to kick start your day..

(Serves 4)
2 apples, cored and chopped
2 kiwi fruit
1 punnet of berries, such as blueberries, raspberries, and strawberries
1 pineapple, peeled, cored, and chopped
2 semi-ripe pears, cored and chopped
12 ounces prunes or other canned fruit in natural juice
Plain yogurt with live bacteria (optional)

Method: Mix all the ingredients together and serve with or without a dollop of yogurt. This keeps for 2 to 3 days, covered tightly, in your refrigerator.

PEANUT BUTTER ON TOAST

Peanuts are an impressive source of protein that can give you a boost to start your day.

Peanut butter — buy peanut butter that doesn't have any added sugar, salt, or palm oil from a whole-food store or farmers' market
Wholewheat toast

Method: What could be simpler – just spread the peanut butter on the toast and you'll be set up for the whole morning.

OATY DIVINE

This dish sets you up for the day, because the oats help balance your blood-sugar levels.

(Serves 1)
⅔ cup oatmeal
⅔ cup mixture of water and milk (oat milk is gorgeous)
1 tablespoon raisins

1 dried fig, chopped with the middle stems removed
½ handful of toasted and chopped almonds

Method: Place the oats and liquid mixture into a heavy-bottomed saucepan over medium heat. Bring to a simmer and stir for 3 minutes before taking the pan off the heat. Add the remaining ingredients and leave to blend for another minute longer. Eat at once while still hot.

BANANA SMOOTHIE
This smoothie provides you with a great vitamin C lift.

(Makes 1 smoothie)
1 banana, peeled
1 kiwi fruit, peeled
1 small apple, cored and quartered
1 pear, cored and quartered
A splash of fruit juice

Method: Place all ingredients into a blender and blend until smooth.

HOMEMADE MUESLI
A perfect way to start the day. This recipe can be stored for up to two weeks in an airtight container.

(Makes 12 servings)
4⅓ cups jumbo rolled oats
1 heaped cup mixed seeds, such as sunflower and pumpkin
1⅓ cups chopped nuts, such as Brazil nuts and almonds
1⅓ cups semi-dried figs cut into quarters
1¼ cup dried apple rings or halves, roughly chopped
1 cup dried cranberries
Plain yogurt or milk to serve

Method: Heat the oven to 375°F. Spread the jumbo oats in a large roasting pan and bake for 15 minutes. Stir in the seeds and continue to bake for 5 minutes longer, or until golden brown.

Tip the oats and seeds into a large bowl and leave to cool completely. Add the nuts and dried fruit and toss all the ingredients together. Transfer to an airtight container for storage.

To serve, soak a portion of muesli in a little yogurt or milk and leave overnight in the refrigerator. It will be ready for breakfast the following morning. Soaking the muesli softens the oats and gives the cereal a lovely creamy texture. If you prefer a crunchy breakfast, however, simply pour cold milk or juice onto your muesli and eat straightaway.

WHOLE GRAIN PANCAKES

(Makes 24 small pancakes)
2 cups wholewheat flour
3 teaspoons baking powder
2 medium eggs
1¼ cups milk
1 teaspoon unpasteurized honey
Dribble of olive oil for cooking

Method: Mix together the dry ingredients. Make a well in the center and add the eggs and the milk. Stir with a wooden spoon incorporating the flour from the sides as you stir and don't worry about the small lumps. Add the honey and stir into the mixture.

Heat a heavy-bottomed non-stick skillet and pour in a few drops of oil and smear them around with some non-stick paper. Pour spoonfuls of batter onto the skillet to form 3-inch pancakes. They will bubble and sizzle. When they look dry around the edges, turn them over. They should have a golden brown color. Place them on a platter and keep them warm with a covered cloth.

Serve with whole fruit (no sugar) jam or my yummy Fig and Apricot Compote (page 158).

BERRY YUMMY

Eat a bowl of your favorite berries with a chopped banana mixed in for a supporting boost of antioxidants and stress-relieving serotonin.

7-DAY PLAN TO BEAT DEPRESSION

From the first day I felt better and by the end of the seven days I felt fantastic.

PENNY LEEDAM, AGED 36

MONDAY

Lunch
TUNA ON WHOLEWHEAT

Nothing beats a scrumptious tuna sandwich to satisfy you at lunchtime. Try this one for the omega-3 boost in the tuna and a shot of folate from the avocado.

(Makes 2 sandwiches)
1 can (6-oz.) tuna in spring water, drained
1 tablespoon mayonnaise made with olive oil
Balsamic vinegar
Lettuce leaves
1 ripe avocado, peeled, stoned and sliced
4 slices wholewheat bread spread with Ace Butter
   (page 86)

Method: Mix the tuna with the mayonnaise and balsamic vinegar to taste. Place the lettuce on 2 slices of bread. Spread the tuna on each slice, then add the avocado slices and top each slice with the remaining bread slices. If you're not eating the sandwiches straightaway, wrap them in foil for freshness.

Supper
A POT OF LOVE
This delicious one-pot meal is a rich source of iron.

(Serves 4)
1 tablespoon olive oil
2 onions, chopped
3 cloves of garlic, crushed
1 teaspoon ground cumin
1 teaspoon curry powder
½ teaspoon ground cinnamon
4 carrots, scrubbed and sliced
½ cup dried green lentils
1 cup long-grain brown rice
2½ cups chicken or vegetable stock
1 apple, cored and diced
4 scallions, sliced
Plain yogurt with live bacteria to serve

Method: Heat the oil in a large saucepan over medium heat. Add the onions, garlic, cumin, curry powder, and cinnamon and fry, stirring often, for about 5 minutes until soft. Stir in carrots, lentils, and rice and continue to fry, stirring, for 1 minute. Pour in stock and bring to a boil, skimming the surface as necessary.

Reduce the heat to low, cover, and leave to simmer for 20 minutes, or until the rice and lentils are tender and most of the liquid is absorbed. Stir in the apple and scallions and continue to simmer, covered, for 5 minutes, or until the scallions are heated through. Serve with a dollop of yogurt.

TUESDAY

Lunch
SOOTHING VEGETABLE SOUP

There is nothing more nurturing than a home-made soup.

(Serves 4)

1 tablespoon olive oil

1 onion, finely chopped

2 cloves garlic, crushed

2½ cups diced vegetables, such as broccoli, bell pepper, carrot, celery, and a sweet potato

1½ cups strained puréed tomatoes (look for 'passata' at an Italian food store)

1¼ cups vegetable stock

Pinch of dried oregano

Ground black pepper to taste

Method: Heat the olive oil in a saucepan over medium heat. Add the onion and stir around for 3 to 5 minutes until the onion is soft, but not brown. Stir in the garlic and diced vegetables, then cover and leave to sweat for a couple of minutes.

Stir in the tomatoes, stock, oregano, and pepper and continue simmering, covered, for 20 minutes until all the vegetables are tender. If you make this the night before, reheat and place into your wide-necked vacuum flask for lunch.

Supper
SWEET POTATO AND CARROT MASH

Serve this with a portion of your favorite lean red meat to give you an added boost of iron.

(Serves 4)

3 cups peeled and chopped carrots

3 cups peeled and roughly chopped sweet potatoes

Knob of Ace Butter (page 86)

10 ounces lean beef or lamb

1 pound broccoli, trimmed and cut into spears

Method: Place the carrots and sweet potato in a saucepan with cold water to cover. Bring to a boil, then reduce the heat and simmer for 10 minutes, or until the vegetables are tender.

Drain the vegetables thoroughly, then return them to the heat for about one minute to remove the excess liquid. Mash the carrots and sweet potatoes together, then add a knob of Ace Butter.

Meanwhile, broil your meat and place your broccoli in a steamer and steam until tender-crisp. Add a touch of Ace Butter to your broccoli and serve at once with the meat and mashed vegetables.

WEDNESDAY

Lunch
PASTA WITH PESTO AND PUMPKIN SEEDS
Loaded with vitamin E and omega-3s to lift your spirits.

8 ounces thin green beans, trimmed
2½ cups dried wholewheat pasta spirals
⅔ cup pumpkin seeds, toasted
For the pesto sauce:
1 clove of garlic, finely chopped
⅔ cup pine nuts
Handful basil, leaves only
⅔ cup freshly grated Pecorino Romano cheese
Extra-virgin olive oil

Method: First make the pesto. Put the garlic, pine nuts, basil, and cheese in a blender and blend until finely chopped. Slowly add olive oil until the pesto has the consistency of coarse sand; set aside.

Meanwhile, bring a large pan of water to a boil. Add the green beans and boil for about 3 minutes, or until tender-crisp. Using a draining spoon, remove the beans from the pan, drain well and set aside. Return the cooking water to a boil, add the pasta and continue boiling for 8 to 10 minutes, or according to the directions on the package.

Just before the pasta is tender to the bite, remove 2 tablespoons of the cooking water and stir it into the pesto. When the pasta is tender, drain it well, then tip into in a large bowl. Add the pesto, green beans, and pumpkin seeds and toss together. Serve at once or set aside and leave to cool completely, then put in a plastic container for transporting to work.

Supper
SLAP-HAPPY MACKEREL AND PAN-ROASTED TOMATOES

The antioxidants in the tomatoes together with the mackerel's omega-3s will help to banish your gloom.

- 3 tablespoons olive oil
- 2 shallots, finely chopped
- 1 pound tomatoes
- 1¼ cups dry white wine
- 4 medium mackerel
- 4 cloves of garlic, peeled
- 3 tablespoons finely chopped fresh parsley
- A pinch of finely chopped fresh sage
- Freshly steamed brown rice to serve

Method: Gently heat a large, heavy-bottomed skillet over medium heat. Add the oil and shallots and fry for 3 minutes, stirring frequently. Place the tomatoes on top of the shallots, cover the skillet, and leave the tomatoes to cook gently for about 10 minutes until soft to the touch. Pour in the wine, place the mackerel on top of the tomatoes, and sprinkle with the garlic. Re-cover the skillet and leave the fish to cook in the steamy sauce for about 10 minutes until they are cooked through and the flesh flakes easily. Stir in the parsley and sage just before serving. Serve with a portion of hot brown rice.

THURSDAY

Lunch
GRIN WITH GARBANZO SALAD

Garbanzo beans have a low-GI factor and provide slow-release energy, which helps balance your sugar levels so you feel good. Eat this yummy salad with gusto!

¾ cup dried garbanzo beans, or 1 can (15-oz.) garbanzo beans, drained and rinsed

3 tablespoons olive oil

2 cloves of garlic, chopped

1 teaspoon cayenne pepper, or 1 fresh red chili, seeded and chopped

2 teaspoons ground cumin

Juice of 1 lemon

Handful of baby spinach leaves

1 tablespoon plain yogurt with live bacteria

1 bunch fresh parsley, chopped

Method: If you are using dried garbanzo beans, soak them overnight in cold water, then rinse and drain. Put them in a saucepan with fresh cold water to cover and bring to a boil. Boil for 10 minutes, then reduce the heat and simmer for 1 to 1 1/2 hours until tender; drain well.

Heat 2 tablespoons of the oil in a skillet over medium heat. Add the garlic, cayenne, and cooked or canned garbanzo beans and stir around for 2 minutes. Stir in the cumin and half the lemon juice and continue cooking until the juices in the pan evaporate. Turn off the heat and stir in the spinach leaves, stirring until they wilt. Stir in the yogurt, parsley, oil and the remaining lemon juice. Eat at once, or leave to cool completely and put in a plastic container for transporting to work.

Supper
EAT AND TWO VEG

The vegetables in this pie help strengthen the nervous system, while the fiber promotes a healthy digestive system.

1½ pounds Idaho potatoes, peeled and cut into chunks
1 small cauliflower, cut into flowerets
1 leek, sliced and rinsed
1 parsnip, peeled, cored, and diced
2 carrots, peeled and diced
3 tablespoons olive oil
1 onion, finely chopped
1 clove of garlic, crushed
1 can (15-oz.) mixed beans, drained and rinsed
1 teaspoon Italian seasoning
2 tablespoons Ace Butter (page 86)
⅔ cup milk or soy milk
¼ cup plus 2 tablespoons wholewheat flour

Method: Heat the oven to 350°F. Bring a large pan of lightly salted water to a boil. Add the potatoes and continue boiling until they are tender. Meanwhile, in a steamer over another pan of boiling water, steam the cauliflower, leek, parsnip, and carrots until tender.

At the same time, heat 1 tablespoon of the oil in a large skillet over low heat. Add the onion and garlic and fry gently for 3 minutes, stirring occasionally, until soft. Stir in the beans and Italian seasoning.

In another pan, place the milk, flour, and remaining 2 tablespoons oil and heat, whisking constantly over medium-high heat, until thick.

When the potatoes are tender, drain them well, add the Ace Butter and a splash of milk, and mash them until fluffy. Mix the vegetables, beans, herbs and milk sauce together in a lightly greased baking dish. Place the mashed potato on top and spread out to cover the surface. Bake for 20 minutes until the topping is golden brown.

FRIDAY

Lunch
TUNA AND GREEN BEAN SALAD

The selenium in the tuna and the folate in the beans will help you feel great.

1¾ cups green beans diagonally sliced
1 tablespoon olive oil
One 10-ounce fresh tuna steak
4 scallions, thinly sliced diagonally
1 cup fresh bean sprouts
1 tablespoon fresh cilantro, chopped
For the dressing:
1 tablespoon low-sodium soy sauce
1 tablespoon olive oil
1 fresh red chili, seeded and finely chopped
Juice of 1 lime
2 teaspoons unpasteurized honey

Method: Cook the beans in boiling water for 3 to 4 minutes until tender-crisp, then drain and cool under cold running water. Drain well and pat dry with paper towels; set aside. Meanwhile, heat the oil in a heavy-bottomed skillet or griddle and cook the tuna for about 4 minutes on each side, or until the tuna is cooked through; set aside to cool.

Put the dressing ingredients in a screw-top jar and shake. Place the beans, tuna, and bean spouts into a bowl, carefully breaking up the tuna. Add the dressing and mix well.

Supper
MUSHROOM-STUFFED BUCKWHEAT CREPES

The selenium in the mushrooms, makes this a perfect supper for a mood lift.

(Makes 10–12 crepes)
1 teaspoon malt vinegar

1 cup milk

1 tablespoon olive oil, plus a little extra for cooking the crepes

1¼ cups dark buckwheat flour

2 medium eggs

For the filling:

2 tablespoons olive oil

1 onion, chopped

1 red bell pepper, cored, seeded, and chopped

1 pound fresh chestnut mushrooms, sliced

2 cloves of garlic, crushed

1 teaspoon paprika

Slug of sherry or brandy (optional)

1 bunch of fresh tarragon, chopped

Method: To make the crepes, add the vinegar to the milk in a mixing bowl and leave for 15 minutes until it curdles. Stir in the 1 tablespoon oil and buckwheat flour, then add the eggs, one at a time, making sure they are worked in thoroughly until a thin batter forms.

Heat a medium skillet or crepe pan over a high heat and use a ball of paper towels to brush the surface very lightly with extra oil. Pour 2 to 3 tablespoons of the batter into the skillet and swirl the pan so the batter spreads out. Leave the crepe to cook for about 1 minute until golden brown on the bottom, then flip it over and cook on the other side. Remove from the pan and keep warm in a low oven while you make more crepes until all the batter has been used. (Layer the crepes with waxed paper to prevent them sticking.)

Meanwhile, to make the filling, heat the oil in another skillet over medium heat. Add the onion and fry, stirring, until soft, but not brown. Add the peppers and mushrooms and continue stirring until they are soft. Stir in all the garlic, paprika, and sherry and simmer until the liquid reduces. Add the tarragon and take the pan off the heat.

To serve, simply divide the filling between the crépes and roll them up. Brown rice is a delicious accompaniment.

SATURDAY

Lunch
AVOCADO, TOMATO AND BABY LEAF SALAD

This is a divine salad for a weekend lunch treat, packed with antioxidants and folate.

3 ripe avocados, peeled, stoned and sliced
6 ripe plum tomatoes, halved and thinly sliced
1 red onion, halved and thinly sliced
Handful of baby lettuce leaves, rinsed and dried
⅔ cup sunflower seeds, toasted
1 bunch of fresh basil, chopped
Shavings of Pecorino Romano cheese to garnish
Dressing:
4 tablespoons extra-virgin olive oil
1 tablespoon balsamic vinegar
2 teaspoons unpasteurized honey
1 small clove of garlic, finely grated

Method: Mix all the salad ingredients, except the Pecorino cheese, together in a large bowl, then arrange on plates. Whisk together the dressing ingredients and pour over the salad. Scatter the Pecorino and serve immediately.

Supper
FRESH MACKEREL WITH SAFFRON

The omega-3-packed mackerel and the calming effect of the saffron will help ease you toward a good night's sleep.

    2 tablespoons olive oil, plus a little extra for the roasting pan
    3 cups sliced potatoes
    4 mackerel, each weighing 6 to 8 ounces
    4 tomatoes, sliced
    1 cup white wine
    1 cup water
    Pinch of saffron
    2 cloves garlic, chopped
    1 small bunch of fresh dill, chopped
    1 lemon, quartered, to garnish
    Green salad to serve

Method: Heat the oven to 400°F. Spread the potatoes on the bottom of a well-oiled roasting pan. Arrange the tomatoes on top and add the mackerel. Mix the saffron with the wine and water and pour the mixture over. Sprinkle in the garlic cloves. Put the pan in the oven and bake for 30 minutes, or until the mackerel is cooked through and flesh flakes easily. Sprinkle with the dill and garnish with the lemon quarters. Serve with a green side salad.

SUNDAY

Lunch
ROAST CHICKEN WITH BRAZIL NUT STUFFING

The Brazil nuts boost your selenium intake – a must for raising your emotional health.

1 chicken, weighing about 3 pounds
1 tablespoon olive oil
Freshly ground black pepper
2 tablespoons sunflower oil
2 potatoes per person, par-boiled
A selection of seasonal vegetables, prepared as necessary and cut into similar-size pieces
1 tablespoon all-purpose flour
2 cups chicken or vegetable stock
Brazil nut stuffing:
3 tablespoons olive oil, plus a little extra for the baking dish
1 large onion, chopped
2 cloves of garlic, chopped
2 cups chopped Brazil nuts
⅔ cup sunflower seeds, toasted
1 bunch of fresh sage, chopped
2 cups fresh coarse wholewheat bread crumbs
2 eggs, lightly beaten

Method: Heat the oven to 400°F. First make the stuffing. Heat the oil in a large skillet over medium heat. Add the onion and fry gently, stirring, for 3 to 5 minutes. Add the garlic and continue frying for 3 minutes longer. Remove the pan from the heat and stir in the Brazil nuts, sunflower seeds, bread crumbs, sage and eggs. Mix well and place into a greased baking dish; set aside.

Place the chicken in a roasting pan, dribble with the 1 tablespoon olive oil, and sprinkle with the pepper. Place into oven and roast for 1 hour, or until the juices run clear when you pierce the thickest part of the thigh with a knife. After 30 minutes, place the potatoes in another pan and dribble with the sunflower oil. Place them in the top of the oven. Also place the dish with the stuffing in the oven.

Prepare your vegetables and put them on to steam 15 minutes before you are due to serve. When the chicken is cooked through, place it on a tray for carving and leave to stand for 10 to 15 minutes. Make your gravy by pouring off the excess fat, then adding the flour to the pan and stirring over low heat for 2 to 3 minutes. Slowly whisk in the stock and bubble the liquid until becomes smooth and thick. Serve immediately. **Cooks' tip:** gravy powder now comes in a low-salt version. This is a quick and easy alternative for making gravy.

Supper
LEFTOVER CHICKEN/TURKEY WITH WARM POTATO SALAD

Potatoes are full of folate, B-vitamins, and vitamin C to aid immunity and help to raise a good mood – a perfect end to the weekend.

For the warm potato salad:
1 pound new potatoes, scrubbed
A generous handful of fresh parsley leaves
½ cup snipped fresh chives
1 teaspoon Dijon mustard
1 tablespoon balsamic vinegar
3 tablespoons olive oil
Freshly ground black pepper
Pickles and relishes to serve

Method: Cook the potatoes in a pan of boiling water until tender. Drain well and place in a serving bowl. Add all the other ingredients while the potatoes are still warm and gently stir together. Serve with your leftover lunch and a selection of pickles and relishes.

7-DAY PLAN TO BEAT STRESS

I was pretty stressed before I started eating this new diet
… Now I have a much better feeling of wellbeing and I'm
learning which foods to eat to keep my stress down.
MALCOLM BAILY, AGED 49

MONDAY

Lunch
GARBANZO STEW WITH LENTILS

A protein-packed lunch to give you all the energy you need to
see you through the afternoon. With the calcium in the
garbanzos helping your stress levels, you should feel good until
suppertime.

- ⅓ cup dried garbanzo beans or 12 ounces canned garbanzo beans
- 2 cups chicken or vegetable stock
- 1 cup lentils
- 1 bay leaf, some thyme and oregano tied together (use the thyme or oregano as string)
- 4 carrots, peeled and finely chopped
- ½ head white cabbage, cored and shredded
- Chapatti or pita bread to serve (optional)

Method: Soak the garbanzo beans in plenty of water to cover
overnight. In the morning, drain the beans and place them in a
pan with 1 cup of water. Bring to a boil and boil hard for 10
minutes, then reduce the heat to low, cover, and simmer for 30
minutes, topping up the water if necessary. Drain the beans
and place into a clean pan with the stock and simmer for 20
minutes or until tender but holding their shape. (If you are
using canned beans, simply drain them and place into a pan
with the stock at this point.)

Add the lentils and the herbs and continue to simmer for 10 minutes. Add the carrots and simmer for a further 10 minutes, or until the carrots are tender-crisp. Add the cabbage and simmer just until it is tender. Season with pepper to taste. Serve with a warm chapatti or pita bread.

Supper
SALMON FISHCAKE WITH TARRAGON

A delicious way to eat omega-3 fats as the sauce from the fish infuses your brown rice and vegetables. If you have more fishcakes than you want, the extras can be frozen for another time.

(makes 4 fishcakes)
8 scallions, finely chopped
1 pound salmon fillets, skinned, if necessary, and diced
Finely grated zest and juice of 2 limes
1 tablespoon fresh tarragon
1 tablespoon olive oil
To serve:
Steamed brown rice
Freshly cooked green vegetable, such as spinach, green beans, or broccoli

Method: Heat the oven to 400°F. Place all the ingredients into a bowl and mix thoroughly. Grease four 4-inch cooking rings and place them on a greased cookie sheet. Divide the salmon mixture between the cooking rings, smoothing the tops. Bake for 15 to 20 minutes until firm and the salmon is cooked through. Serve with brown rice and spinach, green beans, or broccoli.

TUESDAY

Lunch
PASTA SALAD WITH TUNA AND CHERRY TOMATOES

This salad keeps well in a plastic container, so you can take it with you to work.

> 1½ cups dried wholewheat pasta shells
> 12 cherry tomatoes
> 3 tablespoons olive oil
> 4 medium eggs
> 2 cans (8-oz.) butter or lima beans, drained and rinsed
> 1 can (6-oz.) tuna in spring water, drained
> *Dressing:*
> 3 tablespoons olive oil
> 1 teaspoon vinegar or lemon juice
> 1 teaspoon mustard
> 1 teaspoon manuka or other unpasteurized honey
> Fresh herbs, such as chives, parsley, or cilantro, chopped
>   (optional)

Method: Bring a large saucepan of water to a boil. Add the pasta shells and boil for 10 to 12 minutes, or following the directions on the package, until tender to the bite. Drain well, then set aside to cool.

Place the cherry tomatoes in a pan over medium heat with 1 tablespoon of olive oil and heat through until the tomatoes are soft. Take the pan off the heat and set aside to cool. Meanwhile, bring another pan of water to a boil. Add the eggs and boil for exactly 10 minutes. Remove the eggs and place under cold running water to stop the cooking. When the eggs are cool, shell and quarter them.

To make the dressing, whisk the oil, lemon juice or vinegar, mustard, and honey together in the bottom of your serving bowl. Add all the other ingredients and gently toss together.

Supper
COD WITH SWEET POTATOES AND PARSLEY

The magnesium in the cod and the vitamin C in the sweet potato will help replenish you after a busy day.

1 white potato, peeled and cut into ¾-inch chunks
4 small sweet potatoes, peeled and cut into ¾-inch chunks
4 cod fillets, about 5 ounces each
2 tablespoons olive oil, plus a few drizzles for the potatoes
Bunch of parsley, chopped
Juice of 1 lemon
Freshly cooked green vegetable, such as broccoli, green beans, or spinach, to serve

Method: Heat the oven to 400°F. Place the white and sweet potatoes in a roasting pan, drizzle with the olive oil and roast for 45 to 50 minutes until tender.

Meanwhile, cut 4 pieces of foil each large enough to enclose a piece of cod. Place the fish on the foil, then top each with one-quarter of the lemon juice and olive oil and scatter with the parsley. Seal the parcels securely, so no steam can escape, and place on a baking sheet.

After the potatoes have roasted for 30 minutes, place the baking sheet in the oven and leave the fish to cook for 15 minutes. The lemon juice will steam the cod to perfection.

To serve, set the potatoes on a plate and then place the cod with the juice over the potatoes. Complete the meal with a lightly steamed portion of your favorite green vegetable.

WEDNESDAY

Lunch
TURKEY AND BEAN STEW

This stew promotes the tryptophan in your diet, which helps you feel calm and relaxed. If you're at work at lunchtime, prepare this filling stew the night before and then reheat and spoon into your flask the following morning.

3 tablespoons olive oil
1 red onion, chopped
2 red bell peppers, cored, seeded, and sliced
1½ pounds boneless turkey breast halved, skinned and sliced
1½ cups sliced green beans
1 leek, sliced
1 clove of garlic, crushed
1¾ cups vegetable stock
1 bunch of fresh parsley, chopped
Wholeweat bread or roll

Method: Heat the oil in a saucepan over medium heat. Add the red onion and the pepper and sauté for 2 to 3 minutes. Add the turkey and continue sautéing for 5 minutes. Stir in the beans, leek, and garlic and cook for 1 to 2 minutes longer. Add the vegetable stock and bring to a boil. Reduce the heat to low and simmer for 12 to 14 minutes, or until the stock has reduced and the vegetables are tender. Add the chopped parsley, then spoon into a flask for lunch. Be sure to pack a couple of slices of wholewheat bread or a roll to accompany your stew.

Supper
BAKED POTATO WITH HOUMOUS AND AVOCADO SALAD

A simple meal incorporating magnesium-boosting sesame seeds and the copper-enriched avocado — both great for helping to beat stress. (Note the following day's lunch is houmous sandwich – ensure you make enough houmous for both meals.)

1 large Idaho or baking potato, scrubbed and dried
Olive oil (optional)
For the houmous (makes enough for 2 portions):
1 can (15-oz.) garbanzo beans, drained and rinsed
1 clove of garlic, crushed
2 tablespoons tahini sauce (sesame seed paste)
1 tablespoon olive oil
Juice of 1 lemon
Chopped fresh parsley or cilantro
For the avocado salad:
1 tablespoon olive oil
2 teaspoons balsamic vinegar
1 teaspoon honey
1 avocado, peeled, seeded, and sliced
1 handful of spinach leaves, rinsed
1 heart of lettuce, leaves separated and rinsed
1 tablespoon sunflower seeds, toasted

Method: Begin by baking the potato. Heat the oven to 425°F. Use a fork to prick the potato skin all over. If you like crisp skins on your baked potatoes, rub a small amount of oil all over it. Place the potato on a baking sheet and roast for 1 to 1½ hours until it feels very soft and tender when squeezed. (If you are short of time, spear the potato with metal skewers, which conducts heat to the middle so it cooks quicker.)

Meanwhile, put all the ingredients for the houmous in a food processor and blend until almost smooth. If it is too thick, add a few tablespoons extra lemon juice or water; set aside.

To make the avocado salad, put the olive oil, vinegar, and honey in a mixing bowl and whisk together. Add the avocado, spinach, lettuce, and sunflower seeds and gently toss together. To serve, slice the potato open and spoon the houmous on top. Serve with the avocado salad on the side.

THURSDAY

Lunch
WHOLEWHEAT BREAD AND HOUMOUS SANDWICH

This simple lunch provides good complex carbohydrates and a complete protein package.

(Makes 1 sandwich)
2 slices wholewheat bread
Ace Butter (page 86)
Houmous (page 187)
Salad leaves
Toasted pine nuts
Cottage cheese

Method: Spread both slices of bread with Ace Butter. Layer the remaining ingredients on one slice until the sandwich is bursting at the seams, then top with the other slice of bread. Cut in half and wrap in foil.

Supper
SALMON AND SESAME SEEDS WITH SPINACH

This simple salmon dish is rich in omega-3s, which will soothe your muscles and aid a good night's sleep.

4 fresh salmon fillets, skin on, about 6 ounces each
6 tablespoons sesame seeds
2 tablespoons olive oil
Freshly steamed brown rice to serve
For the spinach:
9 ounces spinach leaves, well rinsed
Drizzle of olive oil
Juice of 1 lemon

Method: Heat the oven to 350°F. Roll the salmon fillets in the olive oil and then in the sesame seeds until they are completely covered with the seeds. Place in a roasting pan and roast for 20 minutes. Meanwhile, put the spinach in a skillet with just the water clinging to the leaves and heat for about 3 minutes until it wilts. Drain the spinach well, pressing out all the excess water.

Divide the spinach between 4 plates and drizzle with the olive oil and lemon juice. Place a salmon fillet on top of each portion and serve with hot brown rice.

FRIDAY

Lunch
BROCCOLI AND RICE SALAD

This lunch will help you beat stress with the mix of the slow-releasing, low-GI factor of the rice and the folate in the broccoli.

    2 cups brown long-grain rice
    1¾ pounds broccoli flowerets
    ⅔ cup golden raisins
    1 tablespoon low-sodium soy sauce
    Juice of 1 lime
    1 teaspoon unpasteurized honey
    1¼ cups sunflower seeds, toasted

Method: Steam the rice according to the directions on the package. At the same time, steam the broccoli flowerets. Place the rice and the broccoli into a bowl and, while hot, pour over the remaining ingredients and toss together. Set aside to infuse while the broccoli and rice cool.

Supper
BAKED CHICKEN WITH ZUCCHINI AND TOMATOES

The tomatoes in this dish offer a good source of lycopene, which is full of antioxidants and will help boost you up after a busy day.

    3 tablespoons olive oil
    2 red onions, thinly sliced
    4 boneless chicken breasts (each weighing about 4 ounces), skinned and halved
    6 zucchini, sliced
    1 bunch of fresh basil, chopped
    1 pound tomatoes, sliced

To serve:
Mashed potatoes
Steamed green vegetable, such as broccoli, Savoy cabbage, or green beans

Method: Heat the oven to 400°F. Heat the oil in a heavy-bottomed skillet over medium heat. Add the onions and fry for about 3 minutes until soft. Add the chicken and fry for 3 to 4 minutes longer. Then add the zucchini and stir them around for 1 minute.

Transfer all the ingredients to a large, shallow baking dish, arranging the chicken breast halves in a single layer. Sprinkle the basil over the chicken and then lay the tomato slices on top. Bake, uncovered, for 20 minutes until the chicken juices are clear when you pierce the breasts with a knife.

Serve with mashed potato and steamed green vegetables.

SATURDAY

Lunch
SARDINES IN TOMATO SAUCE ON RYE TOAST
A perfect, quick lunch that you can serve in minutes. This simple dish is full of good carbohydrates, omega-3 fatty acids, and tryptophan — all of which act as de-stressors. This is a great cupboard fallback when you haven't been shopping.

(Serves 1)
1 can (4-oz.) of the best sardines in tomato sauce you can find
2 slices of rye bread, toasted

It's very simple — make a sandwich with the sardines.

Supper
RISOTTO WITH KALE AND LEMON

The kale in this delicious risotto serves up magnesium and calcium, two important minerals to appease your day.

1¼ quarts vegetable stock
4 tablespoons olive oil
1 large red onion, chopped
2½ cups risotto rice
3¾ cups shredded kale
Finely grated zest and juice of 1 small lemon
⅔ cup grated Pecorino Romano cheese

Method: Pour the stock into a saucepan and bring to a simmer over low heat. Gently heat the oil in a large, heavy-bottomed saucepan over medium heat. Add the onion and fry, stirring frequently, for about 3 minutes, or until it is beginning to soften. Add the rice and continue to cook, stirring constantly, for 2 minutes.

Add just enough stock to cover the rice and continue simmering, stirring frequently, until most of the stock has been absorbed. Continue adding the stock, a small amount at a time until it is almost completely absorbed and the rice is just tender; this will take 15 to 20 minutes. The consistency of the risotto should be rich and creamy.

Stir in the shredded kale and continue to simmer, stirring constantly, for 3 minutes. Remove the pan from the heat and stir in the lemon zest and juice and half the cheese. Sprinkle with the remaining Pecorino Romano and serve immediately.

SUNDAY

Lunch
THE SUNDAY ROAST

If we had to discard all our old much-loved meals, life might not be worth living. Don't forgo your traditional Sunday roast meal. Instead, follow this healthy alternative and make it the perfect end to the 7-Day Food Plan.

1 chicken or small turkey weighing about 3 pounds
1 tablespoon olive oil
Freshly ground black pepper
2 potatoes per person, par-boiled
2 tablespoons sunflower oil
A selection of seasonal vegetables, prepared as necessary and cut into similar-size pieces
1 tablespoon wholewheat flour
2 cups chicken or vegetable stock

Method: Heat the oven to 400°F. Place the chicken in a roasting pan and dribble of the olive oil and grind some pepper over it. Place into the oven and roast for 1 hour, or until the juices run clear when you pierce the thickest part of the thigh with a knife. After 30 minutes, place the partly boiled potatoes on another pan and dribble with the sunflower oil. Place them in the top of the oven and continue roasting for 30 minutes longer.

Put the vegetables on to steam 15 minutes before you are due to serve. When the chicken is cooked through, place it on a tray for carving and leave to stand for 10 to 15 minutes. Make your gravy by pouring off the excess fat, then adding the flour to the pan and stirring over low heat for 2 to 3 minutes. Slowly whisk in the stock and bubble the liquid until becomes smooth and thick. Serve immediately.

Cook's tip: gravy powder now comes in a low-salt version. This is a quick and easy alternative when making gravy.

Supper
LEFTOVERS WITH WARM PUY LENTIL SALAD

Earthy lentils ooze magnesium for a healthy nervous system.
Simply serve this protein-rich dish with the leftovers from your
Sunday lunch.

    1 heaped cup green Puy lentils
    2 red onions, 1 halved and 1 finely chopped
    1 carrot, peeled and halved
    2 tablespoons balsamic vinegar
    6 tablespoons extra-virgin olive oil
    Salad leaves, rinsed and dried
    9 ounces ripe tomatoes, cut in half
    1 bunch fresh parsley, chopped

Method: Rinse the lentils and put in a saucepan with the
halved onion, carrot, and enough cold water to cover. Bring to a
boil, then reduce the heat, cover, and simmer for 25 minutes,
or until the lentils are tender. Remove the pan from the heat
and leave to stand for 5 minutes, by which time the water
should be almost completely absorbed. Remove the onion and
carrot and tip the lentils into a mixing bowl.

Mix the vinegar and olive oil and add it to the lentils. Add
the chopped red onion and mix thoroughly. Arrange the salad
leaves and tomatoes on individual plates, then spoon the lentil
mixture into the middle each and sprinkle with parsley. Serve
immediately with your leftover roast chicken. Delicious!

7-DAY PLAN TO FIGHT CHRONIC FATIGUE

I had been feeling worn down and fed up for about a year but now I am paying attention to my food and I haven't felt this good for years.

HANNAH LEADER, AGED 47

MONDAY

Lunch
CARROT AND ORANGE SOUP

A good way to get a blast of carotenoids and antioxidants, which enhance immunity and can help your body fight the persistent tiredness and flulike symptoms.

    3 tablespoons olive oil
    6 carrots, peeled and sliced
    1 potato, peeled and diced
    2½ cups vegetable stock
    1 orange, zest and juice only
    2 cloves of garlic, chopped
    1½ tablespoons fresh cilantro, chopped
    Wholewheat bread or rolls to serve

Method: Heat the oil in a saucepan over medium heat. Add the carrot and potato and fry, stirring occasionally, for 2 minutes. Pour in the stock, along with the orange zest and juice and leave to simmer for 10 minutes, or until the carrots are tender. Add the garlic and blend until smooth. Serve with a sprinkling of cilantro and wholewheat bread or rolls.

Supper
LAMB PATTIES WITH GREEK-STYLE YOGURT

Both lamb and plain yogurt contain quantities of vitamin B12 that might help reduce with the muscle ache that comes with chronic fatigue.

(Makes 6 patties)

1 pound very lean, good-quality ground lamb
2 large carrots, peeled and grated
1 small onion, finely chopped
2 cloves of garlic, crushed
1 cup chopped mushrooms
2 teaspoons tomato paste
1 cup fresh mixed-grain or wholewheat bread crumbs
1 green chili, seeded and finely chopped
1 tablespoon roughly chopped fresh mint
1 tablespoon roughly chopped fresh parsley
1 tablespoon roughly chopped fresh cilantro
1 egg
Olive oil for brushing the baking sheet
For yogurt:
⅔ cup plain yogurt with live bacteria
¼ cucumber, chopped
1 tablespoon chopped fresh mint
To serve:
Green salad
Steamed brown rice

Method: Heat the oven to 400°F. Place all the ingredients for the burgers together in a bowl and mix well. Divide into 6 patties. (If you wish, you can freeze them at this point.) Place the burgers on a greased baking sheet and bake for 20 minutes.

Meanwhile, to make the yogurt, simply mix all the ingredients together.

Serve the patties with the yogurt on the side, a green salad, and a portion of steamed rice.

TUESDAY

Lunch
RED CABBAGE SALAD

The enzymes in the energy-boosting red cabbage will help you to stop flagging when you're only halfway through the working day. This salad is moist and sumptuous. Enjoy a large plateful for a filling lunch.

- ⅔ cup dried cranberries, halved
- 6 tablespoons orange juice
- 1 small red cabbage, about 1½ pounds, cored and finely chopped
- 2 tablespoons vinegar
- 6 tablespoons walnut oil
- A handful of freshly chopped fresh tarragon
- 2 sweet dessert apples, cored and chopped
- ⅓ cup roughly chopped Brazil nuts

Method: Soak the dried cranberries in the orange juice in a small bowl for about an hour. Whisk the vinegar, oil, and tarragon together in a serving bowl. Add all the remaining ingredients and mix well. Toss the cranberries.

Supper
STUFFED PEPPERS WITH YOUR FAVORITE FRESH FISH

Red bell peppers are full of vitamins A, C, and E, as well as antioxidants, which are great for aching joints.

For the peppers:
6 tablespoons olive oil
2 medium onions, chopped
4 cloves of garlic, chopped
1½ cups cooked long-grain rice
2 large tomatoes, seeded and finely chopped
1⅓ cups black olives, pitted and chopped
1 tablespoon chopped fresh cilantro
4 red bell peppers, halved, cored, and seeded
Warm pita bread to serve
For the fish:
4 fresh fish, such as mackerel or bass, drawn and rinsed
4 tablespoons white wine or lemon juice

Method: Heat the oven to 425°F. Gently heat the oil in a skillet over medium heat. Add the onion and garlic and fry for a few minutes, stirring, until soft. Stir in the cooked rice, tomatoes, olives, and fresh cilantro and continue stirring for a further few minutes. Place the pepper halves onto a greased baking sheet and divide the rice mixture into them; set aside

Meanwhile, cut 2 pieces of foil large enough to enclose the fish. Place a fish in the centre of each piece of foil, add 1 tablespoon wine or lemon juice to each, then close the package sealing it tightly so no steam escapes during cooking. Place the fish packages on the baking sheet, then put it into the oven for 20 minutes until the fish is cooked through and the peppers are tender.

WEDNESDAY

Lunch
ENERGIZING CRUDITÉS

Let the enzymes of this gorgeous raw-food lunch integrate into your body and help give you a midday energy buzz.

Crudités, as much as you want of:
Peeled and sliced carrots
Sticks of celery
Slices of green and red bell peppers
Small flowerets of broccoli
Oat crackers
Houmous (page 187) to serve

Method: Make the houmous, following the directions on page 187. Cover and chill until required, then place in a plastic container for transporting together with your crudités in a separate bag. You don't even need silverware for this meal!

Supper
STUFFED CHICKEN WITH MASHED PARSNIPS

A good source of protein, potassium, and fiber, all of which help to build the body's strength.

For the chicken:
4 boneless chicken breast halves, skinned
Handful of spinach leaves
5 ounces goat's cheese, crumbled
12 green olives, pitted and chopped
2 cloves of garlic, crushed
3 tablespoons olive oil
1 cup water and/or white wine
Green beans, topped and tailed, steamed, to serve
For the mashed parsnips:
6 parsnips, peeled, cored, and chopped
3 medium potatoes, peeled and chopped
Dribble of olive oil
1 bunch of fresh parsley, chopped

Method: Heat the oven to 400°F. Make a lengthwise slit in the chicken breast halves and open each one like a book. Place several spinach leaves, one-quarter of the cheese, olives, and garlic, and a dribble of olive oil in each. Place in a roasting pan and pour in the liquid.

Place the pan in the oven and roast for 30 minutes. Meanwhile, place the parsnips and potatoes in a saucepan of boiling water and continue to boil until soft. Drain the vegetables well and mash with a dribble of olive oil. Throw in the parsley just before serving. Steam the green beans for 5 minutes until tender and serve on the side.

THURSDAY

Lunch
FAVA BEAN SALAD
The high level of vitamin B5 in the humble fava bean makes this salad a brilliant support against tiredness and stress.

4 cups frozen or shelled fava beans
1½ cups cooked, wholewheat pasta
3 tablespoons olive oil
2 small onions, roughly chopped
2 cloves of garlic, roughly chopped
2 zucchini, sliced
1 cup vegetable stock
1 can (15-oz.) crushed tomatoes
Small bunch of fresh sage leaves, roughly chopped
Wholewheat bread to serve

Method: Put the beans in a pan of boiling water and cook until just tender. At the same time, in another pan of boiling water, cook the pasta for 10 to 12 minutes, or following the directions on the package, until it is tender to the bite. Drain both and set aside.

Heat the olive oil in a large saucepan over low heat. Add the onions and garlic and fry, stirring occasionally for about 3 minutes. Add the zucchini and continue to fry for a few minutes longer until soft. Add the stock and tomatoes with their juices and continue simmering until the mixture is slightly reduced, no more than 10 minutes. Stir in the fava beans and return to a boil, then reduce the heat and simmer 5 minutes longer, or until the beans are tender. Mix in the cooked pasta and sage. Serve straightaway, although this is just as delicious as a cold salad.

Supper
SEARED TUNA WITH ARUGULA AND CHILI

Vitamin B12 deficiency can result in fatigue and anemia, so let this gorgeous tuna dish bolster you up.

> 4 fresh tuna steaks, about 4 ounces each
> About 6 tablespoons olive oil
> 2 teaspoons honey
> Large pinch of dried chili flakes (optional)
> 1 bunch of arugula leaves, rinsed and dried
> 2 cans (15-oz.) crushed tomatoes
> 1 lemon
> *To serve:*
> Boiled new potatoes
> Steamed broccoli flowerets

Method: Rub a little of the oil and half the honey over the tuna steaks and sprinkle with the chili flakes. Lay the arugula leaves on a plate and squeeze the lemon over them together with a drizzle of oil. Heat a large skillet with the remaining oil and honey and sear the tuna steaks for 2 minutes on each side. Stir in the tomatoes and their juice and simmer, uncovered, for 7 minutes until the tomatoes reduce slightly. Place the tuna steaks on top of the arugula leaves, with the tomato sauce spooned over.

FRIDAY

Lunch
AZUKI BEAN STEW

Azuki beans are power-packed with nutrients to help your body release the energy you need from your food.

Olive oil
2 onions, chopped
4 cloves of garlic, finely chopped or crushed
2 medium leeks, rinsed, halved lengthways, and thickly sliced
2 large carrots, peeled and chopped
3½ cups mushrooms cut into chunks unless very small
1 tablespoon paprika
1 teaspoon cayenne pepper, or to taste
1 tablespoon low-sodium soy sauce
2 tablespoons tomato paste
2 cans (15-oz.) crushed tomatoes
1 bunch fresh parsley, chopped
1½ cups dried azuki beans, soaked overnight and cooked for 30 minutes (save the cooking liquid)

Method: Sauté the onions in the oil until softened and starting to brown. Add the garlic, leeks, carrots and mushrooms, and cook for another 5 minutes, until starting to soften. Mix in the paprika and stir for another minute or so. Add all the remaining ingredients except for the parsley, plus half the aduki beans' liquid to half-cover the ingredients.

Stir well, cover and simmer for about 30 minutes, stirring occasionally and adding more cooking liquid if it gets too dry. Season with the parsley and serve with mashed potatoes or place in a wide-necked flask for fast food 'on the go'.

Supper
MACKEREL WITH ROASTED FENNEL

The fennel aids your digestion and helps your body to get the nutrients it needs, while the mackerel offers omega-3 fats, proven to aid fatigue.

- 4 medium bulbs of fennel, trimmed and thickly sliced
- 1 medium red onion, roughly chopped
- 6 tablespoons olive oil
- Juice of 2 lemons
- 4 mackerel, drawn
- 2 bunches of your favorite mixed fresh herbs, such as parsley, dill, tarragon, and/or basil
- 4 cloves of garlic, peeled
- 3 tablespoons bottled capers, drained
- Fresh mixed salad to serve

Method: Heat the oven to 400°F. Place the fennel, onion, olive oil, and lemon juice in a roasting pan and roast for 30 minutes. Meanwhile, open the cavity of the mackerel and stuff with the herbs, garlic, and capers.

Place the mackerel on top of the fennel mixture (after it has roasted for 30 minutes) and put the dish back into the oven for 20 minutes longer, or until the mackerel is cooked through and the flesh flakes easily. The mackerel will infuse with the fennel to make an exquisite meal. Serve with a green salad.

SATURDAY

Lunch
SARDINES ON TOAST

A wonderful way to get another boost of omega-3s, while also getting a dose of tomato lycopene, which is packed with antioxidants to help maintain energy levels.

2 slices wholewheat bread, toasted
1 can (3.75-oz.) sardines in tomato sauce

Method: You can either heat up your sardines or leave them cold, which ever your preference is. Spoon them and the tomato juice over the hot toast.

Supper
RATATOUILLE WITH FRIED SHALLOTS

A deficiency in vitamin B3 can cause fatigue and depression; get a blast of this wonderful vitamin from the zucchini in this recipe.

1 tablespoon olive oil
2 red onions, chopped
8 zucchini, chopped
1 cup dry red wine
2 cloves of garlic, crushed
1 can (15-oz.) crushed tomatoes
2 ounces tomato paste
1 bunch of fresh basil, chopped
Steamed brown rice to serve
For the fried shallots:
6 shallots, thinly sliced
¼ cup wholewheat flour
6 tablespoons sunflower oil

Method: Heat the oil in a skillet over medium heat. Add the red onions and fry, stirring frequently, for 2 to 3 minutes. Add the zucchini and continue stirring for 2 to 3 minutes. Stir in the red wine, garlic, tomatoes with their juices, and the tomato paste and bring to a boil. Leave to reduce for 3 to 4 minutes. Add the chopped basil and keep warm. Meanwhile, dust the shallots with the flour. Heat the oil in a saucepan over high heat. Add the shallots and fry for 2 minutes, or until they are brown. Place on top of the ratatouille and serve with steamed brown rice.

SUNDAY

Lunch
ROAST LAMB WITH GARLIC AND ROSEMARY

Lamb contains significant levels of protein, zinc, riboflavin, and vitamin B12, all of which act as body warriors to help build a strong immune system and fight fatigue.

1 bunch of fresh or dried rosemary
1 leg of lamb, weighing about 6¾ pounds
4 cloves of garlic, sliced
4 tablespoons olive oil
A selection of seasonal vegetables, prepared as necessary, and cut into similar size pieces
For the gravy:
¾ cup beef brown stock
3 cloves of garlic
1-inch piece of cinnamon stick
7 tablespoons dry red wine
2 tablespoons olive oil
2 teaspoons wholewheat flour
2 potatoes per person, par-boiled
Dribble of sunflower oil

Method: Heat the oven to 400°F. Place the rosemary in a roasting pan and put the leg of lamb on top. Cut some nicks in the joint and stuff the pieces of garlic into the cuts. Dribble the olive oil over the lamb and roast for about 1½ hours, or until the meat juices run faintly pink when pierced. Remove the lamb from the pan and leave it to stand while making the gravy.

After the lamb has been in the oven for 30 minutes, place the potatoes in another roasting pan and dribble with the sunflower oil. Place in the top of the oven.

Meanwhile, steam the vegetables for the final 15 minutes while the lamb roasts.

Put the brown stock, garlic cloves, and cinnamon stick in a saucepan over low heat and bring to a simmer. Put the liquid in the roasting pan that contained the lamb. Place the roasting pan over medium heat. Pour in the red wine, stirring well to lift any sediment from the bottom of the pan, then strain and discard the rosemary. Pour into a clean saucepan and bring to a boil. Mix the oil and flour together and quickly whisk into the boiling gravy to slightly thicken. Simmer for 3 to 4 minutes and serve with the lamb.

Supper
LEFTOVERS WITH CARROT AND KOHLRABI SALAD
Kohlrabi is a lesser-known vegetable, somewhere in between a cabbage and a turnip, but contains a high amount of sulforaphane, a powerful component in beating fatigue. If you can't find kohlrabi then simply replace with spinach and reap the rewards of its iron by helping to prevent the symptoms of energy-sapping anemia.

- 2 large carrots, peeled and grated
- 2 kohlrabi, peeled and chopped (if unavailable, use 9 ounces spinach leaves, rinsed)
- 4 tablespoons olive oil
- 4 teaspoons cumin seeds
- Juice of 1 lemon

Method: Simply mix all the salad ingredients together and leave them to infuse for 30 minutes before serving. Place the salad next to slices of lamb from lunch.

INDEX